Learning Disabilities
and Mental Health

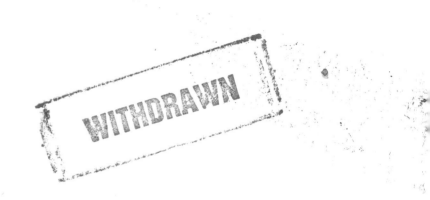

Learning Disabilities and Mental Health

A Nursing Perspective

Raghu Raghavan and Pradip Patel

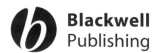

Blackwell
Publishing

© 2005 by Blackwell Publishing Ltd

Editorial offices:
Blackwell Publishing Ltd, 9600 Garsington Road, Oxford OX4 2DQ, UK
  Tel: +44 (0)1865 776868
Blackwell Publishing Inc., 350 Main Street, Malden, MA 02148-5020, USA
  Tel: +1 781 388 8250
Blackwell Publishing Asia Pty Ltd, 550 Swanston Street, Carlton, Victoria 3053, Australia
  Tel: +61 (0)3 8359 1011

First published 2005 by Blackwell Publishing Ltd

Library of Congress Cataloging-in-Publication Data
Raghavan, Raghu.
Learning disabilities and mental health: a nursing perspective/Raghu Raghavan and Pradip Patel.
    p. ; cm.
Includes bibliographical references and index.
ISBN-13: 978-1-4051-0615-3 (pbk. : alk. paper)
ISBN-10: 1-4051-0615-8 (pbk. : alk. paper)
1. Learning disabled–Mental health.   2. Learning disabled–Nursing.   3. Psychiatric nursing.
[DNLM: 1. Mental Disorders–nursing.   2. Community Mental Health Services.
3. Learning Disorders–complications.   4. Mental Disorders–complications.]
I. Patel, Pradip.   II. Title.
RC394.L37R337 2005
362.2'0425–dc22
2005003366

ISBN-10: 1-4051-0615-8
ISBN-13: 978-1-4051-0615-3

A catalogue record for this title is available from the British Library

Set in 10/12.5pt Palatino
by Graphicraft Limited, Hong Kong
Printed and bound in India
by Replika Press Pvt Ltd, Kundli

The publisher's policy is to use permanent paper from mills that operate a sustainable forestry policy, and which has been manufactured from pulp processed using acid-free and elementary chlorine-free practices. Furthermore, the publisher ensures that the text paper and cover board used have met acceptable environmental accreditation standards.

For further information on Blackwell Publishing, visit our website:
www.blackwellpublishing.com

We wish to dedicate this book to our parents and to all people with learning disabilities and mental health issues

Contents

Foreword

John Turnbull
Director of Nursing and Performance, Oxfordshire Learning
Disability NHS Trust

There can be little doubt that nurses working with people with learning disabilities are more confident than they have ever been as they go about fulfilling their main purpose, which is to support individuals in order to lead healthier and more satisfying lives. Whatever the setting, one of the hallmarks of learning disability nurses has been their ability to apply a breadth of knowledge and experience to meet people's needs and aspirations. However, learning disability nurses are increasingly becoming recognised for the depth of their expertise and their capacity to apply this in more specialist and complex circumstances. One example of this is their work with people with learning disabilities who have mental health needs.

For this reason, I hope that this comprehensive and timely publication will support nurses in order to develop their practice in this crucial area and help others to understand the role of nurses better. In my brief contribution to this book I cannot hope to add substantially to the reader's knowledge except to reflect on my personal experience of working with people with mental health needs. Apart from feeling distinctly 'out of my depth' at times, I can remember drawing upon personal qualities such as patience and compassion. Compassion for another's distress and suffering is an aspect of nursing values that is perhaps not automatically associated with learning disability nursing. However, I found it to be a powerful motivator in keeping me focused on the issues that were important to the individuals, as well as a stabilising force, in overcoming the setbacks. I also found that supporting people with learning disabilities and mental health needs taught me what could be achieved through a good quality relationship with a person. Some learning disability nurses bemoan the lack of a 'technology' in supporting people with learning disabilities. I think there is plenty of room for a more traditionally scientific approach, but the quality of relationships with individuals must remain the foundation of our approach. For this reason I make no apologies for seeing learning disability nursing as the purest form of nursing.

Whereas this book will demonstrate how far practice has developed in working with people with mental health needs, nurses should remember that there are still several challenges to be met. For example, mental health is only just achieving greater prominence in the public health agenda. Also, the National Health Service's involvement in the specialist support of people with learning disabilities is still far from enthusiastic, in spite of the *Valuing People* White Paper (Department of Health 2001). Finally, despite the very laudable principle of encouraging the use of mainstream services, it is worth noting that most of the gains in terms of supporting people with learning disabilities and mental health problems have originated from specialist learning disability services. Whatever the solution to these issues, we surely cannot stray too far off the mark by remaining faithful to the needs and aspirations of people with learning disabilities.

Reference

Department of Health (2001) *Valuing People: A New Strategy for Learning Disability for the 21st Century.* London: The Stationery Office.

Acknowledgements

We wish to thank all people with learning disabilities, their families, carers and professionals in the field of learning disability who have helped us to conceptualise the essence of this book through our practice and consultations. The idea for this book developed from our experiences of the difficulties faced by people with learning disabilities, their families and carers in accessing appropriate help and services in meeting their emotional needs. Of particular importance is the continuous struggle of these people and service providers in confronting health inequalities in mainstream health and social care.

We wish to acknowledge the help of Julie Snowden in shaping the chapters on learning disability nursing and professional and legal issues, and Vicky Bliss for contributing to the section on solution focused therapy. Our thanks also go to Beth Knight, Amy Brown, Magenta Lampson and Shahzia Chaudhri from Blackwell Publishing. We gratefully acknowledge the support of our families (Sudha, Vivek, Anand, Julie and Jennifer) in helping us to focus on the task.

We are truly grateful to people with learning disabilities who helped us to formulate case examples to highlight the theory and practice.

Raghu Raghavan
Pradip Patel

Chapter 1

Introduction

Introduction and aims of the book

The changing patterns of care and the movement away from institutions to community living have laid to rest the myth that the psychological problems suffered by those with learning disabilities were the result of institutional-isation alone and that living in the community would somehow 'remove' or 'cure' such problems. In fact community living has resulted in additional stressors, for example, negative attitudes, social exclusion, increased exposure to alcohol and illicit drugs and vulnerability to abuse or exploitation. Such stressors, when combined with the limited coping and problem-solving skills that a person with learning disability often has, is likely to result in problems in day-to-day life and mental heath issues. It is evident that many mental health disorders often go unrecognised due to the phenomenon of diagnostic overshadowing, that is, the assumption that mental disorder and learning disability are mutually exclusive categories rather than overlapping.

It is now generally accepted that people with learning disabilities may also suffer from mental disorders seen in the general population, such as anxiety, depression, schizophrenia, dementia and personality disorder (Eaton and Menolascino 1982; Campbell and Malone 1991). The superimposition of mental health disorders in people with learning disabilities is known as *dual diagnosis*. However, this term is also commonly used in acute mental health care to identify people with both a mental health disorder and a drug or alcohol problem. In this book we have followed the former definition, and use the term *people with dual diagnosis* to specify people with learning disabilities who also experience mental health disorders.

The estimated prevalence of dual diagnosis ranges from 10 to 80%, but there is a consensus that 30 to 40% of people with intellectual disabilities experience a range of mental health disorders during their lives. For most of the common mental health disorders, the estimated prevalence in people with learning disabilities is far higher than in the general population. Many learning disability nurses and a significant number of mental health nurses are in daily contact with this group, but their complex needs are not well understood by these health care professionals. This may be attributed to a lack of appropriate knowledge, skills and confidence in working with people, as well as a general lack of understanding within mainstream mental health services about how learning disability mental health liaison nurses can contribute positively to the co-ordination and the therapeutic delivery of mental health care for this population.

We think that nurses working in the field of learning disability and mental health should have a sound knowledge base for shaping and enhancing their clinical practice. With this in mind, this book aims to explore issues concerning the mental health of people with learning disabilities, including:

- The prevalence, nature and manifestation of mental health disorders in people with learning disabilities
- Issues and models of detection and diagnosis of mental health disorders in people with learning disabilities
- Needs assessment for therapeutic intervention and services
- Pharmacological and psychosocial interventions
- The learning disability nurse as therapist
- Professional and legal issues to enhance safe practice, taking into consideration the vulnerability of people with learning disabilities
- Policy and service perspectives

Developing evidence-based practice is a key theme of this book and we have attempted to focus the issues and practice-based evidence on the aforementioned themes. However, the lack of a significant systematic evidence base poses a challenge for nurses and other health and social care practitioners working in this field. The real challenge here is to reflect on the rich and diverse ways of working with people with dual diagnosis in order to develop a model of practice-based evidence.

In this book, we explore the role of the learning disability nurse as a therapist in working with people with dual diagnosis. We believe that through the consolidation of the evidence base for assessment, intervention and services, learning disability and other nurses will be able to utilise this knowledge in planning and developing therapeutic nursing practices when providing person-centred care for people with leaning disabilities and mental health disorders.

The structure of this book

People with dual diagnosis present unique challenges to health professionals, in terms of both diagnosis and the provision of appropriate therapeutic services. Considering the nature of dual diagnosis, people with a learning disability and mental health disorder will require a mixture of generic and specialist services. The White Paper *Valuing People: A New Strategy for Learning Disability for the 21st Century* (Department of Health 2001) indicates that the National Service Framework (NSF) for mental health applies to all people of working age and therefore is applicable to people with learning disabilities (Department of Health 1999). From an ideological perspective, people with learning disabilities who experience mental health disorders are expected to access mainstream mental health services for mental health care and support. The challenge is for mainstream health and social care services (including mental health services) to provide therapeutic support and help for people with learning disabilities that respects individuality, choice and independence. Both learning disability and mental health services have a long history and we have seen the implementation of a number of Government polices aimed at improving the services for this population. This gives a clear vision of how services are anticipated to develop in the future. The concepts of learning disability and mental health and mental health disorders are explored in Chapter 2.

For many years, professionals from various fields have debated whether people with learning disabilities could become emotionally disturbed or mentally ill (Scheerenberger 1987). People with mild learning disability were thought by carers to be 'worry free', and people with severe learning disabilities were considered to have no feelings (Nezu 1994). Studies published in the last two decades document a high prevalence of mental health disorders in people with learning disabilities (Eaton and Menolascino 1982; Reid 1989; Bouras and Drummond 1992). Such mental health problems can often go unrecognised, as shown by Reiss in his studies on the phenomenon of 'diagnostic overshadowing' (Reiss et al. 1982; Spengler et al. 1990; Sovner and Pary 1993). This refers to instances in which the presence of learning disability decreases the diagnostic significance of an accompanying mental health disorder. Hence, there is a tendency to underdiagnose mental health disorders in people with learning disabilities, because some of the debilitating emotional problems may appear less significant when compared with the effects of learning disability. The extent of overlap between challenging behaviour and mental health disorder has also been the subject of many debates, and its impact on detection and diagnosis of mental health disorders in people with learning disabilities is very confusing. Nurses and other health and social care practitioners need to understand the prevalence, nature and manifestation of mental health disorders in people with learning disabilities in order to conceptualise the issues of providing therapeutic care, and this is explored in Chapter 3.

There is considerable debate about how mental health problems manifest in those with different degrees of learning disability. There is a broad consensus that in those with mild learning disability, such disorders present in a more typical way and can be diagnosed by applying criteria that are used in the general population using *International Classification of Diseases-10* (World Health Organization 1993) and the *Diagnostic and Statistical Manual of Mental Disorders (DSM-IV)* (American Psychiatric Association 1994) with minor modifications, for example as suggested in *DC-LD* (*Diagnostic Criteria for Psychiatric Disorders for Use with Adults with Learning Disabilities/Mental Retardation* (Royal College of Psychiatrists 2001). There is much more debate about how such disorders manifest in those who have severe to profound learning disabilities. Here mental health problems often present in atypical, more individualised forms, as behavioural disorders, and assessment requires a more qualitative, case study approach using person-centred planning models and behavioural approaches such as functional analysis.

Unrecognised mental health problems in those with learning disabilities can have a major effect on their general well-being, personal independence, productivity and quality of life, as well as impacting on family and other carers. The combination of learning disabilities and mental ill-health can also give rise to stigmatisation and prejudices which lead to social exclusion. Differential diagnosis of challenging behaviour and mental health disorder may have serious consequences in understanding the therapeutic needs of this particular population and developing effective ways of working. We explore the issues concerning assessment and diagnosis in Chapter 4.

Due to the complex and confusing nature of dual diagnosis, the form and types of needs of people with learning disability who also experience mental health disorders are not well understood by service providers and professionals in this field. It is argued that people with dual diagnosis have intricate needs, which are often poorly identified, and such people are shifted between mental health and learning disability services in fruitless attempts to obtain adequate therapeutic services (Menolascino 1989). This calls for a systematic process of identifying needs and providing appropriate interventions to meet these needs. With this in mind, we explore the concept of need and its assessment for people with dual diagnosis in Chapter 5.

People with learning disabilities make up a diverse group and often have additional physical and sensory disabilities or epilepsy which makes them more vulnerable to suffering from a mental health disorder. A number of factors, broadly divided into developmental/biological, psychological and social, combine to lead to mental disorder in a given individual. Such factors can either increase the risk of mental disorder or in some circumstances protect the person from mental health problems. For example, a person with learning disabilities who has a valued lifestyle with supportive consistent carers would be less vulnerable to additional unpredictable stressors such as bereavement than someone who is living in deprived circumstances with inconsistent carers or support.

Providing therapeutic care to address the mental health needs of people with learning disabilities requires in-depth understanding of the biopsychosocial dimensions of learning disability. Learning disability nurses by virtue of their training and experience play a significant role in health assessment, health facilitation and co-ordination of care in the multidisciplinary environment. The contribution of learning disability nurses in caring for people with dual diagnosis is explored in Chapter 6 using the framework of therapeutic nursing.

Our knowledge base of therapeutic interventions for people with dual diagnosis is slowly expanding. People with dual diagnosis require psycho-pharmacological as well as psychosocial interventions in the treatment of mental health disorders. We have considered various types of medication used in treating mental health disorders and its application to people with learning disabilities. We have also explored the advances in psychopharmacology, with the introduction of new forms of drugs with minimal side effects. Too often, medication is the sole intervention used in mental health disorders. We believe that the psychosocial interventions such as cognitive behaviour therapy, behavioural and psychotherapeutic approaches are equally as important as medication. Psychopharmacological and psychosocial interventions are explored with available evidence base in Chapters 7 and 8.

Care for people with dual diagnosis needs to be undertaken with professional integrity, respecting the individuality, rights and choices of people. We need to understand the issues of consenting to assessment and treatment and how we can help people with learning disabilities make the right choice. It also involves risk taking and hence it is important for nurses and other health and social care practitioners to have a sound knowledge base in risk and risk assessment. These important issues along with mental health legislation are explored in Chapter 9.

Recent strategic documents such as the National Service Framework (NSF) for mental health disorders and the *Valuing People* White Paper on service development for those with learning disabilities recommend that mainstream psychiatric services should be accessible to those with learning disabilities. When such services are inappropriate, for example due to lack of expertise or vulnerability of clients with learning disability when admitted to a general psychiatric ward, appropriate back-up specialist services should be available. There is continuing debate about how capable mainstream mental health services are in meeting the diverse needs of those with learning disabilities. The role of specialist services and the policy directions for service development are explored in Chapter 10.

To provide therapeutic care, we need to conduct a thorough assessment of the problems and needs of people. These call for the use of structured assessment processes using standardised screening tools, interview schedules, rating scales and checklists. A range of instruments in assessing the mental well-being and behaviour of people with learning disabilities is considered in Appendix 1.

Appendix 2 concludes the book by covering some genetic syndromes related to mental health.

This book will introduce a range of concepts relating to the mental health needs of people with intellectual disabilities. This will include the nature, prevalence, causes and manifestation of mental health disorders in this population. The question of how nurses should assess the needs of people with intellectual disabilities and offer needs-led therapeutic services is addressed. This book will provide an in-depth knowledge base for learning disability and mental health nurses from an evidence-based perspective, which should have an impact on their clinical practice and in service development.

References

American Psychiatric Association (1994) *Diagnostic and Statistical Manual of Mental Disorders (DSM-IV)*. Washington DC: APA.

Bouras, N. and Drummond, C. (1992) Behaviour and psychiatric disorders of people with mental handicaps living in the community. *Journal of Intellectual Disability Research*, **36**, 349–357.

Campbell, M. and Malone, R.P. (1991) Mental retardation and psychiatric disorders. *Hospital and Community Psychiatry*, **42**, 374–379.

Department of Health (1999) *National Service Framework for Mental Health. Modern Standards and Service Models*. London: Department of Health.

Department of Health (2001) *Valuing People: A New Strategy for Learning Disability for the 21st Century*. London: The Stationery Office.

Eaton, L.F. and Menolascino, F.J. (1982) Psychiatric disorders in the mentally retarded: types, problems and challenges. *American Journal of Psychiatry*, **139**, 1297–1303.

Menolascino, F.J. (1989) Model services for treatment/management of the mentally retarded–mentally ill. *Community Mental Health Journal*, **5**, 145–155.

Nezu, A.M. (1994) Mental retardation and mental illness. *Journal of Consulting and Clinical Psychology*, **62**, 4–5.

Reid, A.H. (1989) Psychiatry and mental handicap: a historical perspective. *Journal of Mental Deficiency Research*, **33**, 363–368.

Reiss, S., Levitan, G.W. and Szyszo, J. (1982) Emotional disturbance and mental retardation: diagnostic overshadowing. *American Journal of Mental Deficiency*, **86**, 567–574.

Royal College of Psychiatrists (2001) *DC-LD (Diagnostic Criteria for Psychiatric Disorders for Use with Adults with Learning Disabilities/Mental Retardation)*. London: Gaskell Press.

Scheerenberger, R.C. (1987) *A History of Mental Retardation: A Quarter of Century Practice*. London: Paul H. Brookes.

Sovner, R. and Pary, R.J. (1993) Affective disorders in developmentally disabled persons. In: J.L. Matson and R.P. Barrett (Eds) *Psychopathology in the Mentally Retarded*. Boston: Allyn and Bacan.

Spengler, P.M., Strohmer, D.C. and Prout, H.T. (1990) Testing the robustness of the diagnostic overshadowing bias. *American Journal on Mental Retardation*, **95**, 204–214.

World Health Organization (1993) *The ICD-10 Classification of Mental and Behavioural Disorders. Diagnostic Criteria for Research*. Geneva: WHO.

Chapter 2
Learning disability and mental health

People with learning disabilities and people with mental illness are marginalised citizens in our society. The fields of learning disability and mental health have a long history and are constantly at the forefront of new policy initiatives for promoting equality, choice and inclusion. This chapter explores the concepts of learning disability and mental health as two distinct fields and then discusses the mental health needs of people with learning disabilities. The mental health needs of children and young people with learning disabilities are often ignored and their plight is highlighted in this chapter. Our societies and communities are increasingly becoming multicultural in composition and therefore the issues of culture, ethnicity, learning disability and mental health are also discussed.

Key themes

- Nature and definition of learning disability
- Nature and definition of mental health
- Mental health needs of children and young people with learning disabilities
- Cultural diversity, learning disability and mental health
- Current issues and policy frameworks for mental health and learning disability services

What is learning disability?

The term *learning disability* has been in use in the UK since 1991, before which time the term *mental handicap* was used to describe people with significant developmental delay which results in arrested or incomplete achievement of the 'normal' milestones of human development. The prevalence estimate of learning disability in England is based on service estimates and not on a total population study. It is estimated that there are about 210 000 people with severe or profound learning disabilities in England, and about 1.2 million people with mild or moderate learning disability (Department of Health 2001).

In Scotland it is estimated that there are around 120 000 people with learning disabilities (Scottish Executive Health Department 2000).

In *Valuing People* (Department of Health 2001) learning disability includes the presence of:

- a significantly reduced ability to understand new or complex information, to learn new skills (impaired intelligence); along with
- a reduced ability to cope independently (impaired social functioning);
- which started before adulthood, with a lasting effect on development.

The term learning disability should not be confused with *learning difficulties*, as the latter is more concerned with problems of learning in educational settings. However, many people with learning disabilities would classify themselves as having learning difficulties and wish to be associated with this term. According to the Education Act 1996, a child having learning difficulty will require special educational provision. The Education Act 1996 defines that a child has a learning difficulty if one of the following applies:

- He or she has a significantly greater difficulty in learning than the majority of children of his/her own age.
- He or she has a disability that either prevents or hinders him/her from making use of educational facilities of a kind generally provided for children of his/her age in schools within the area of the local education authority.
- He or she is under the age of five and is, or would be if special educational provision were not made for him/her, likely to experience severe learning difficulties when of or over that age.

The definition also includes 'statemented children' who may have behaviour problems. (This refers to written statements of educational needs which the local education authority is legally required to meet.) Many people working in learning disability services tend to use the terms learning disability and learning difficulty interchangeably to identify people with learning disabilities, which may be confusing.

In the rest of Europe, the USA, Canada and Asia, the term *mental retardation* is widely used. However, in recent years we have seen the use of terms such as *developmental disability* and *intellectual disability*. In the USA professionals use the term *people with mental retardation* as opposed to calling them mentally retarded. The American Association on Mental Retardation (AAMR) defines mental retardation as:

'the substantial limitations in present functioning of an individual. It is characterized by significantly sub-average intellectual functioning, existing concurrently with related limitations in two or more of the following applicable adaptive skills areas, such as communication, self-care, home living, social skills, community use, self-direction, health and safety, functional academics, leisure and work.'

The AAMR states that 'mental retardation manifests itself before age 18' (Luckasson et al. 1992).

Policies and services

The ideologies and the push for better services for people with learning disabilities over the last three decades have influenced the vision of a better quality of care in the community. The model of an 'ordinary life' perspective for people with learning disabilities was offered by the *Report of the Committee of Inquiry into Mental Handicap Nursing and Care* [Department of Health and Social Security (DHSS) 1979]. This suggested a range of service developments from a '. . . belief in the primacy of "normal" life style . . .', which aimed towards '. . . a decent and dignified life for mentally handicapped people.' The Jay report (DHSS 1979), *The All-Wales Strategy* (AWS) *for the Development of Services for Mentally Handicapped People* in Wales (Welsh Office 1983) and the King's Fund Centre (1980) position paper *An Ordinary Life* have all contributed to the strategic thinking and framework for a community-based service model. Throughout the 1980s, the King's Fund Centre document acted as a focus for the conceptualisation, design and implementation of ordinary community services for people with learning disabilities (Felce 1996).

The major leap from 'devalued' client group and segregated services to a trend-setting 'service user' status with equal rights to generic services in the community was established through major social engineering processes by stressing the theme of consumerism. Rapley and Ridgway (1998) argued that such a new construction emerged from the Second Report of the Social Services Committee of the House of Commons *Community Care: With Special Reference to Adult Mentally Ill and Mentally Handicapped People* (Social Services Committee 1985). This report concluded that, with sufficient financial and human resources, local authorities – rather than hospitals or other providers – could and would provide adequate services for people with learning disabilities. The review of community care policy by the Griffiths report (1988) consolidated the role of market forces in emphasising the 'mixed economy of care', stressing the need for 'cost-effectiveness' and 'value for money' services. The Griffiths report also stressed the value of a multiplicity of provision of services for consumers with choice, flexibility and innovation.

As a result, the care of people with learning disability was becoming increasingly based in ordinary community settings, with the expectation of increased participation and take-up of generic services in the late 1980s and early 1990s. The agenda of community-based services for people with learning disabilities was further reinforced by the then Health Secretary Stephen Dorrell in 1994, in a key speech outlining the ideological scene with three key value statements (*MENCAP Speech*, Department of Health 1994):

(1) That people with learning disabilities – of whatever degree – are entitled to be treated with the same respect and dignity as everyone else. They are people whose views and wishes, as well as their relationships and friendships, must be taken seriously and respected at all times.
(2) That people with learning disabilities should have their health and social care assessed on an individual basis, and not be offered predetermined sets of services because of ill-considered or outdated notions of what people with learning disabilities actually need or should be satisfied with.
(3) That people with learning disabilities have the same rights in relation to statutory services as anyone else. This includes the right of access to both primary and secondary health care as well as the right to have their needs for social care assessed. To secure this in reality means that any special difficulties they may have in enjoying equality of access and assessment must also be recognised and assessed.

In the reforms following the implementation of the National Health Service (NHS) and Community Care Act (Department of Health 1990), local authorities were entrusted with the lead statutory responsibility for assessing the care needs of people with learning disability. The MENCAP speech by Stephen Dorrell in June 1994 outlined the 'social care' model for people with learning disabilities. This suggests that local authorities should plan and arrange a wide range of home-based, day and residential services by contracting them from the voluntary and private sector. An important aspect of this speech is the need to move away from the reliance and trust placed primarily on 'facilities' to 'a system of care and support which can be trusted'. This is a vision 'of a system which disabled individuals and their parents or carers can trust to respond flexibly and sensitively to the needs and preferences which themselves may change significantly over time' (Department of Health 1994). Indeed, this notion of care has taken learning disability services to new realms of service planning and delivery, which is reflected in our current diversity of service provisions.

The notion of social care also acknowledges that even people with severe or profound learning disabilities do not need to spend their lives in hospital simply by virtue of their disability. It is suggested that local authorities must assess each individual's needs and within the resources plan a package of services. This should be aimed at ensuring that the person with learning disability receives care tailored to his/her needs in the setting that offers most scope for the individual's development and well-being. This is a marked shift in the planning and delivery of services for people with learning disabilities, and indeed poses a major challenge to the thinking of professionals in both health and social services. The introduction of the NHS and Community

Care Act 1990 made the purchasers and providers of all health care services and the health authorities obliged to address the health needs of every individual within their district and this included people with learning disabilities.

The complex and challenging needs of people with learning disabilities received much attention in the 1990s. First, the Mansell report *Services for People with Learning Disabilities and Challenging Behaviour or Mental Health Needs* (Department of Health 1993) suggested that service planning and delivery for people with learning disability with challenging behaviour and/or mental health needs should be highly individualised to meet the widely differing needs of these people. The Mansell report placed a heavy emphasis on commissioners and service providers to develop locally based services for people with challenging behaviour. The *Signposts for Success in Commissioning and Providing Health Services for People with Learning Disabilities* (NHS Executive 1998) highlighted the health requirements of people with learning disabilities and the need to access primary care services in the first instance. This document also emphasised the complex needs involved in challenging behaviour and mental health and advocated the development of a range of appropriate services to meet the needs of people with learning disabilities.

The Government White Paper *Valuing People: A New Strategy for Learning Disability for the 21st Century* (Department of Health 2001) in England reflects these themes and is based on the premise that people with learning disabilities are people first and they should therefore use generic services for health care. The vision outlined in this document is based on four key principles: rights, independence, choice and inclusion. These comprise the following:

- *Legal and civil rights*: commitment to enforceable civil rights for disabled people in order to eradicate discrimination in society. People with learning disabilities have the right to a decent education, to grow up, to vote, to marry and have a family, and to express their opinions, with help and support to do so when necessary. All public services will treat people with learning disabilities as individuals, with respect for their dignity, and challenge discrimination on all grounds including disability. Full protection of the law is provided when necessary.
- *Independence*: commitment in promoting the independence of people with learning disabilities. While people's individual needs differ, the starting presumption should be one of independence, rather than dependence, with public services providing the support needed to maximise this. Independence in this context does not mean doing everything unaided.
- *Choice*: like other people, people with learning disabilities want a real say in where they live, what work they should do and who will look after them. However, for many people with learning disabilities these are currently unattainable goals. We believe everyone should be able to make choices. This includes people with severe and profound disabilities, who, with the right help and support, can make important choices and express preferences about their day-to-day lives.

- *Inclusion*: being part of the mainstream is something most of us take for granted. Inclusion means enabling people with learning disabilities to do ordinary things, make use of mainstream services and be fully included in the local community.

In Scotland, *The Same As You? A Review of Services for People with Learning Disabilities* (Scottish Executive Health Department 2000) document identifies seven principles, which will form the backbone to the development of services for people with learning disabilities. They are as follows:

(1) People with learning disabilities should be valued. They should be asked and encouraged to contribute to the community in which they live.
(2) People with learning disabilities are individuals.
(3) People with learning disabilities should be asked about services they need and be involved in making choices about what they want.
(4) People with learning disabilities should be helped and supported to do everything they are able to do.
(5) People with learning disabilities should be able to use the same local services as everyone else, whenever possible.
(6) People with learning disabilities should benefit from specialist, health and educational services.
(7) People with learning disabilities should receive services that take account of their age, abilities and other needs.

The mental health care of people with learning disabilities tends to be based in specialist inpatient units. *The Same as You?* document stresses the need to access mainstream mental health services.

In Wales, a report to the National Assembly for Wales entitled *Fulfilling Promises: Proposals for a Framework for Services for People with Learning Disability* (Learning Disability Advisory Group 2001) proposed that people with learning disabilities of all ages should have:

- A right to similar good health as other people, to have their general health needs met by primary health care services, and to receive equity of access to secondary and specialised health provision as appropriate.
- A right to expect treatment form health care workers who have received adequate training in the recognition and provision of appropriate care.
- A right to skilled specialist help to diagnose and, if required, manage and provide appropriate support for particular conditions, such as autistic spectrum disorders.

The *Fulfilling Promises* document states that people with learning disability and mental health needs should be able to access local mental health services.

In Northern Ireland, services for people with learning disability are seen as part of learning disability hospital and community services. The mental health needs of people with learning disabilities continue to include hospital treatment for people with mild learning disability in specialist services, and the community-based treatment model is yet to be developed.

In England, the White Paper *Valuing People* has set a number of objectives, which form the backbone of transforming the learning disability services in England. By emphasising a value base and the identification of clear objectives (11 sets of objectives), this strategy document helps to place the person with learning disabilities and his or her carers at the centre of seeking ordinary services. The Government stresses the importance of working in partnership with people with learning disabilities, their carers and all agencies that provide services for these people, by setting up local learning disability partnership boards. The health improvement plan advocated in the strategy involves the use of mainstream health and social care services, an identified health action plan and the appointment of health facilitators to the local community team caring for people with learning disabilities. In many areas of the UK this is currently being implemented, and in the next few years we will be able to see and evaluate how these systems are working in the best interests of people with learning disabilities and their carers.

Mental health and mental illness

It is estimated that one in six people of working age in the general population has a mental health problem (Department of Health 1999). From a lay perspective, the terms *mental health* and *mental illness* may be used to indicate the presence of a psychological imbalance in the normal functioning of an individual in society (Box 2.1). What is confusing in the literature and in the health care setting is the use of these two terms interchangeably to indicate mental illness. The notion of mental health is not just the absence of mental illness, but a positive outlook on life and living, which involves the mind–body relationship, our inner thoughts, feelings and behaviour and a balanced psychological and social functioning in society. The physical and social environment of a person, his or her culture and belief systems and in some cases religious beliefs are significant factors in understanding mental health.

Definitions of mental health

'Mental health is the capacity to live life to the full in ways that enable us to realise our own natural potentialities, and that unite us with rather than divide us from all other human beings who make up our world.' (Guntrip 1964, p. 25)

'Mental health is a label, which covers different perspectives and concerns, such as the absence of incapacitating symptoms, integration of psychological functioning, effective conduct of personal and social life, feelings of ethical and spiritual well-being and so on.' (Kakar 1984, p. 3)

Box 2.1   Facts on mental illness.

The World Health Organization states that:

- About 450 million people worldwide are affected by mental, neurological or behavioural problems at any given time. These problems are expected to increase considerably in the years to come.
- Mental problems are common to all countries, cause immense human suffering, social exclusion, disability and poor quality of life. They also increase mortality and cause staggering economic and social costs.
- One in every four persons going to health services has at least one mental, neurological or behavioural disorder. Most often these are neither diagnosed nor treated.
- Cost-effective treatments for most disorders do exist and, if used correctly, could permit affected persons to be functioning members of the community. Yet, in most countries there are major barriers to both the care and the reintegration of people with mental disorders.
- Setbacks include the lack of recognition, awareness and action. Policy makers, insurance companies, health and labour policies, and the public at large all discriminate between physical and mental problems. This discrimination leads to stigma against people who need help.

According to the Department of Health (1995), mental health consists of the follwing four key capacities of an individual:

(1) The ability to develop psychologically, emotionally, intellectually and spiritually
(2) The ability to initiate, develop and sustain mutually satisfying personal relationships
(3) The ability to become aware of others and to empathise with them
(4) The ability to use psychological distress as a development process, so that it does not hinder or impair further development

Generally speaking, all individuals have their ups and downs in their mental functioning, but not everybody develops a mental illness. So there may be distinct biological, social and cultural stress factors that may trigger mental illness. It is very difficult to define what is mental illness, and in the majority of cases the presence of mental illness is often associated with manifestation of abnormal behavioural symptoms. The Mental Health Act 1983 defines mental disorder as the 'arrested or incomplete development of mind, psychopathic disorder and any other disorder or disability of mind'. According to this Act, there are four categories of mental disorder: mental illness, severe mental impairment, mental impairment and psychopathic disorder. For more detail see Chapter 9, p. 177.

It is generally believed that the field of psychiatry is concerned with mental illness or mental disorder, which implies that psychiatric disorders are disorders of the mind and not disorders of the body. Philosophically speaking, neither minds nor bodies develop illnesses. Only people (or, in the wider context, organisms) do so, and when they do, mind and body, psyche and soma, are usually involved (Kendel 2001). In his discussion on the distinction between mental and physical illness Kendel argues that 'it may not be possible to identify any characteristic features of either the symptomatology or the aetiology of so-called mental illnesses that consistently distinguish them from physical illness' (p. 491). He concludes that the distinction between mental and physical illness is ill-founded and incompatible with contemporary understanding of the disease; it is also damaging to the long-term interests of patients themselves. According to Kendel, the idea that mental illness is less 'real' than those of physical disorders with tangible local pathology is confusing in the context of the complex mind–body relationship.

Children and young people

Children and young people with learning disabilities and their families experience many difficulties in receiving adequate therapeutic services. It is estimated that there are about 1.7 million pupils with special educational needs in schools, and nearly 250 000 of these pupils have statements of special educational needs (Department of Health 2001). *Count Us In: The Report of the Committee of Inquiry into Meeting the Mental Health Needs of Young People with Learning Disabilities* (Foundation for People with Learning Disabilities 2002) estimates that 8.7 million people in the UK are between 13 and 24 years of age. Children and young people with learning disabilities experience the added burden of the stresses and strains of growing up. They face many additional barriers of lack of information and access to health care facilities and negative experiences such as labelling and isolation.

Recent studies report a high prevalence of psychopathology in children and young people with learning disabilities, ranging from 30 to 50% (Hoare et al. 1998; Cormack et al. 2000; Emerson 2003). School-leavers with learning disabilities often face difficulties in making a smooth transition from school to college and/or employment. The choices available to many young people after leaving school are very limited and for many do not exist. Transition to adulthood and adult services is a stressful phase for young people and their families. By law (in England), young people with learning disabilities should have a transition plan worked out at school in consultation with the young person and his/her family. Heslop et al. (2002), in their study of transition, found that only few youngsters with learning disabilities had transition plans and many had actually left school without a plan. They found that many young people had very little involvement in planning their future. The lack of a clearly worked out transition plan and co-ordination between children's services and adult services puts many young people and their families under enormous stress during this phase. There is also a lack of information of the various options available after leaving school for young people and their families. These and other socio-economic factors such as poverty, unemployment and poor housing put young people with learning disabilities at increased risk of developing mental health disorders.

Ethnicity, mental health disorders and learning disability

Britain is increasingly seen as a multicultural society, with the promotion of cultural diversity seen as a slogan in public services such as health and education. In fact, it is fashionable to say that we live in a multicultural society, but the hidden realities and experiences of many people from diverse cultures is one of marginalisation and racism. The McPherson Report (Home Office 1999) into the murder of a young black person in south London showed officially that public institutions in British society were institutionally racist and called this *institutional racism*.

Although people from black, minority and ethnic (BME) backgrounds have been present in large numbers in the UK since the Second World War (people from Africa, South Asia, the Caribbean, Ireland, Poland and the Ukraine), research in the last two decades has shown that many of these people face inequalities, discrimination and disadvantage in our society. People from BME groups form a significant part of the UK population, about 4.6 million people (7.9% of the population) in the 2001 census (**www.statistics.gov.uk**). We are currently seeing a steady rise in numbers of people from diverse cultures and religious beliefs in Europe and other western countries such as the USA and Canada, and it is important that we understand the prevalence of the spectrum of learning disabilities, its meaning in their cultures and its consequences in minority communities in order to adequately meet their needs.

It is estimated that the prevalence of severe learning disability in South Asians aged between 5 and 32 years is up to three times higher than in other communities (Azmi et al. 1997). Prevalence estimates in other minority communities in the UK are not well documented.

There is a lack of information of the prevalence of mental illness and/or challenging behaviour in young people with learning disabilities from the South Asian community. However, clinical practitioners and educational staff report that a number of young people from this community do experience emotional difficulties, which may be expressed through challenging behaviour. The overlap of challenging behaviour and mental illness in young people from the South Asian community often clouds the detection and diagnostic process and thus access to appropriate services. Emerson and Robertson (2002) argue that South Asian families supporting young people with learning disabilities at home often do so in the face of considerable adversity – poverty and poor housing and carers having little support from outside the family. Young people from Asian communities have limited social and recreational activities and limited social networks (Hatton et al. 2002). All these trigger factors place young people with learning disabilities from the South Asian community at increased risk of developing psychological disturbances, challenging behaviour and/or mental illness. However, there is only limited service access and utilisation by these young people. Cultural diversity issues are explored in relation to service perspectives in Chapter 10.

Mental health of people with learning disabilities

The belief that people with learning disabilities are not susceptible to mental illness is no longer a valid statement as the policy documents clearly indicate the need for service to focus on the mental health needs of this population. The White Paper *Valuing People* states that most psychiatric disorders are common in people with learning disabilities and that the National Service Framework (NSF) for Mental Health, which applies to all adults of working age, is applicable to people with learning disabilities. The *Valuing People* document stresses the integration of the Care Programme Approach (CPA) and care management. In line with the seven standards identified in the NSF for mental health, the *Valuing People* document sets out the seven areas of attention for people with learning disabilities in order to meet their mental health needs.

The past three decades have seen a major shift in the model of learning disabilities from a dependent and medical model to that of an ordinary citizen with rights of equal access to and use of ordinary community facilities. The closure of the majority of long-stay institutions in the UK has led to the expansion of wide-ranging patterns of services in the voluntary and independent sectors. We have seen a steady shift of services from the statutory sector to the independent and private sectors, with a heavy emphasis on individualised services to meet the needs of people with learning disabilities. We are also seeing the integration of learning disability services as part of primary care and some of the specialised mental health services for people with learning disabilities merging with mainstream mental health services. Services for people with learning disabilities in the NHS tend to focus on specialised services such as health assessment and interventions, behaviour and mental health services.

The changes in the service structure and patterns of service delivery have had a major impact on the key professionals working with people with learning disabilities, especially learning disability nurses. Learning disability nursing is one area that has had to adapt to constant changes in Government policy and the resulting service changes due to the closure of long-stay institutions as a result of the community care legislation and the health and social care model of service provision. A sound knowledge base of the mental health aspects of people with learning disabilities is essential for learning disability and mental health nurses to work with this population.

References

Azmi, S., Hatton, C., Emerson, E. and Caine, A. (1997) Listening to adolescents and adults with intellectual disabilities from South Asian communities. *Journal of Applied Research in Intellectual Disabilities*, **10**, 250–263.

Cormack, K.F.M., Brown, A.C. and Hastings, R.P. (2000) Behavioural and emotional difficulties in students attending schools for children and adolescents with severe intellectual disability. *Journal of Intellectual Disability*, **44**, 124–129.

Department of Health (1990) *The National Health Service and Community Care Act*. London: HMSO.

Department of Health (1993) *Services for People with Learning Disabilities and Challenging Behaviour or Mental Health Needs* (Chairman: Professor J. Mansell). London: HMSO.

Department of Health (1994) *Stephen Dorrell's MENCAP Speech/Statement on Services for People with Learning Disabilities*, 25 June. London: HMSO.

Department of Health (1995) *The Health of the Nation: A Strategy for People with Learning Disabilities*. London: HMSO.

Department of Health (1999) *Facing the Facts: Services for People with Learning Disabilities: A Policy Impact Study of Social Care and Health Services*. London: Department of Health.

Department of Health (2001) *Valuing People: A New Strategy for Learning Disability for the 21st Century*. London: The Stationery Office.

Department of Health and Social Security (DHSS) (1979) *Report of the Committee of Inquiry into Mental Handicap Nursing and Care*. Vols I and II, Cmnd 7468-I, 7468-II (Chairman: Mrs. P. Jay). London: HMSO.

Emerson, E. (2003) Prevalence of psychiatric disorders in children and adolescents with and without intellectual disability. *Journal of Intellectual Disability Research*, **47**, 51–58.

Emerson, E. and Robertson, J. (2002) *Future Demand for Services for Young People with Learning Disabilities from South Asian and Black Communities in Birmingham*. Lancaster: Institute of Health Research, Lancaster University.

Felce, D. (1996) Changing residential services: from institutions to ordinary living. In: P. Mittler and V. Sinason (Eds) *Changing Policy for People with Learning Disabilities*. London: Cassell.

Foundation for People with Learning Disabilities (2002) *Count Us In: The Report of the Committee of Inquiry into Meeting the Mental Health Needs of Young People with Learning Disabilities*. London: Foundation for People with Learning Disabilities.

Griffiths, R. (1988) *Community Care: Agenda for Action*. London: HMSO.

Guntrip, H. (1964) *Healing the Sick Mind*. London: Allen and Unwin.

Hatton, C., Akram, Y., Shah, R., Robertson, J. and Emerson, E. (2002) *Supporting South Asian Families with a Child with Severe Disabilities: A Report to the Department of Health*. Lancaster: Institute of Health Research, Lancaster University.

Heslop, P. et al. (2002) *Bridging the Divide: What Happens for Young People with Learning Difficulties and Their Families?* Kidderminister: British Institute of Learning Disabilities.

Hoare, P., Harris, M., Jackson, P. and Kerley, S. (1998) A community survey of children with severe intellectual disabilities and their families: psychological adjustment, carer distress and the effect of respite care. *Journal of Intellectual Disability Research*, **42**, 218–227.

Home Office (1999) *The Stephen Lawrence Inquiry. Report of an Inquiry by Sir William McPherson of Cluny*. CM4262-I. London: The Stationery Office.

Kakar, S. (1984) *Shamans, Mystics and Doctors: a Psychological Enquiry into India and its Healing Traditions*. London: Unwin.

Kendel, R.E. (2001) The distinction between mental and physical illness. *British Journal of Psychiatry*, **178**, 490–493.

King's Fund Centre (1980) *An Ordinary Life*. London: King's Fund Centre.

Learning Disability Advisory Group (2001) *Fulfilling Promises: Proposals for a Framework for Services for People with Learning Disability*. Cardiff: National Assembly for Wales.

Luckasson, R., Coulter, D.L. and Polloway, E.A. (1992) *Mental Retardation: Definition, Classification, and Systems of Supports*. Washington DC: American Association on Mental Retardation.

NHS Executive (1998) *Signposts for Success in Commissioning and Providing Health Services for People with Learning Disabilities*. London: Department of Health.

Rapley, M. and Ridgway, J. (1998) 'Quality of life' talk and the corporatisation of intellectual disability. *Disability and Society*, **13**, 451–471.

Scottish Executive Health Department (2000) *The Same as You? A Review of Services for People with Learning Disabilities*. Edinburgh: The Stationery Office.

Social Services Committee (1985) *Community Care: With Special Reference to Adult Mentally Ill and Mentally Handicapped People*. Second Report of the Social Services Committee of the House of Commons, Session 1984–5. London: HMSO.

Welsh Office (1983) *The All-Wales Strategy for the Development of Services for Mentally Handicapped People*. Cardiff: Welsh Office.

Chapter 3

Nature, prevalence and manifestation of dual diagnosis

This chapter will explore the issues of mental health and policy framework for mental health services in general. It is important for carers and professionals involved in providing services for people with learning disabilities to have a broad understanding of the nature, manifestation and prevalence of and confusions surrounding the problems relating to behaviour and mental illness. The aim of this chapter is to discuss the knowledge base of mental health aspects of people with learning disabilities using the available evidence.

Key themes

- Nature, prevalence and causes of mental health disorders in children and adults with learning disabilities
- Nature of behaviour problems or challenging behaviour and its overlap with mental health disorders

The nature of mental health disorder

In the wider general population, the detection and diagnosis of mental disorder is more difficult compared to a physical disorder or illness due to lack of objective physical signs of illness or specific diagnostic tests. ICD-10 is a standard classification of illnesses and disorders published by the World Health Organization. *The ICD-10 Classification of Mental and Behavioural Disorders* states that 'disorder' is not an exact term, and 'it is used to imply the existence of a clinically recognizable set of symptoms or behaviour associated in most cases with subjective distress and with interference of physical functions' (World Health Organization 1993). The diagnosis of mental disorder is based on the objective and accurate collection of clinical data by history taking and examination of the mental state. This requires good verbal communication by the client, adequate time for assessment and often corroborative information from a number of different sources. A more accurate diagnosis requires longitudinal

information in addition to cross-sectional interview data, with experts interpreting these data to make a judgement about the presence or absence of a
disorder. Sometimes co-morbidity can occur, for example major depression
has a high co-morbidity with other disorders, particularly anxiety disorders
and substance misuse (Gelder et al. 2001), and it is often difficult to decide
which is primary and which is secondary.

The boundaries between normality and disorder are often blurred, especially
in the early stages of the disorder or in the milder forms, thus making the task
of detection more complicated. The disorder may become clearer over time;
hence initially a more tentative diagnosis may have to be made. Mental disorder is associated with changes in the psychological, social and occupational
functioning of the individual concerned. In a person with learning disability
such functioning may already be low due to the learning disability itself, thus
making it more difficult to define the additional decline in functioning that is
due to the mental disorder. Limited verbal communication makes the process
of diagnosis and detection even more difficult, requiring undue reliance on
information from carers and third parties as well as observations and interpretation of associated behavioural change. This makes the process of diagnosis
using criteria derived from the general population less reliable and valid,
especially in those with severe and profound mental retardation. It is suggested
that the reader keeps these issues in mind when thinking about research on
the prevalence of mental disorders in those with a learning disability.

The nature and manifestation of dual diagnosis

People with learning disabilities have a high risk of developing additional
mental health problems that can go unrecognised and have a major effect on
general well-being, personal independence, productivity and quality of life, as
well as impacting on family and other carers. The last three decades have seen
a surge in the reporting of mental health disorder in people with learning
disabilities. Research reports suggest that these people experience the full range
of psychosis, neuroses, personality disorders, behaviour disorders and adjustment reactions (Phillips and Williams 1975; Eaton and Menolascino 1982).
However, the real nature and the manifestation of mental health disorder in
this population are still open to debate and confusion. This raises two main
questions:

(1) Does the manifestation of mental health disorder in this population differ
     significantly to that of the general population? If this is true then how
     applicable are diagnostic criteria derived from the general population to
     this group. Furthermore, the population of people with learning disabilities
     is a heterogeneous group. Thus the criteria for the general population
     may be more applicable to those with mild or moderate learning disabilities
     rather than those with more severe and profound learning disabilities.

How do we decide when the criteria are applicable? What do we do for those for whom the criteria are not applicable?

(2) If people with learning disabilities are more vulnerable to mental disorder, what could be the possible contributing factors? Current knowledge relating to increased vulnerability to mental illness is based on assumptions from research studies and requires systematic examination of the existing literature and the views and opinions of people with learning disabilities, their family carers, professionals and support workers.

The prevalence studies discussed will throw much needed light on some of these factors, but the real impact of mental health disorder in people with learning disabilities warrants closer examination. The main types of mental health disorders reported in this population include anxiety disorders, affective disorders, schizophrenia, dementia and personality disorders. The real impact of mental health disorders in people with learning disabilities is still not well understood by health care professionals working in this field. Reiss (1993) was one of the first people to shed light on this matter; he focused on the level of functioning of people with learning disabilities, which is the first to be affected at the onset of mental health disorder (Fig. 3.1).

Reiss suggests that people without any learning disabilities function above the minimum level needed for independent living and hence psychopathology must be very severe to suppress functioning to a level requiring hospitalisation. On the other hand, people with mild learning disabilities function only marginally above the minimum level required for independent living, and hence, less severe mental disorders can result in residential placement or

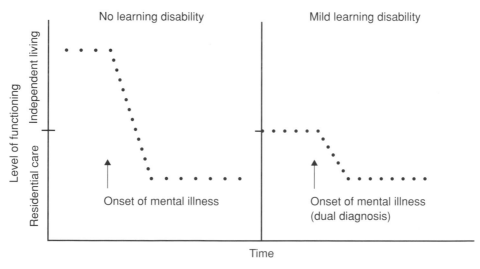

Fig. 3.1 Impact of mental health disorder in the general population and in people with learning disabilities (redrawn from Reiss 1993).

hospitalisation. It is important to have a thorough understanding of the level of functioning of the person, that is their likes and dislikes, overall skills and abilities, nature and types of personal interactions, motivation, interests and patterns of daily living. In people with severe and complex learning disabilities, as the onset of mental illness is often not clearly observable, we may be able to gauge the onset of mental illness by the lack of interest in general or unusual behaviour patterns or the decline in the overall level of functioning. The story of Jackie helps us to explain the need to focus on the skills and abilities of the person with learning disabilities in detecting mental health disorders.

> Jackie is a 45-year-old woman with severe learning disabilities, living in a staffed group home with five other people with a range of learning disabilities. Jackie is able to walk around the house, but uses a wheelchair when out of the house. Jackie has good eye contact with carers and smiles when carers talk to her. She has no speech and uses only few Makaton signs to communicate her needs and wishes. Over the past 6 months some staff members have been reporting that Jackie is looking sad all the time and is increasingly spending her time in her room. She is showing behaviours such as spontaneous screaming and hitting other people in the group home. She is reluctant to go out and gets very agitated when staff attempt to take her out.
>
> Staff only took real notice of Jackie's mood and behaviour when these problems became unmanageable for them in the setting. The staff are demanding that she be moved to some other place, as they are not able to care for her in the group home. The psychiatrist saw her. When asked about Jackie's mood and behaviour over the past 6 months, the staff provided some verbal account of her personality. The staff were unable to report clearly the time when Jackie started to show a change in her mood and behaviour. If there had been a baseline assessment of Jackie's skills and behaviour, and if staff had been knowledgeable enough to understand and detect the symptoms at the onset, it would have been possible to identify the trigger factors and also to provide appropriate interventions prior to the worsening of the situation.

Prevalence studies

This section will explore the range of prevalence studies of mental health disorders in people with learning disabilities. In epidemiological studies, the rate at which a disorder is present in a given population is classified into: (1) *incidence rates*, which represent the number of new cases of a disorder reported within a time period, and (2) *prevalence rates*, which represent the total number of cases with a disorder.

Professionals working in the field of learning disabilities or related disciplines have conducted a large number of studies in an effort to identify the prevalence of mental illness in people with learning disabilities, predominantly in the USA, UK and Scandinavia. For the purpose of discussion, these studies are ordered according to the type of study, and fall into the following groups:

- Representative samples of population – studies based on a random sample of a total population of people with learning disabilities in a geographical area
- Referred samples to psychiatrists – studies based on number of people referred to psychiatrists for psychiatric investigation
- Hospital or institutional settings – studies based on a survey of people with learning disabilities admitted to or staying in a hospital or treatment unit

Studies based on representative samples

These studies indicate a higher prevalence of mental illness in people with learning disabilities than in people without any learning disabilities. The prevalence estimates in people with mild, moderate and severe classifications provide an inconsistent and confusing picture. The methodological aspects adopted and the use of different types of instruments for screening, detection and diagnosis may have contributed to this process. In order to identify true prevalence estimates it is important to interview people with learning disabilities and their carers using structured diagnostic measures rather than relying on case note information.

Study	Prevalence of psychiatric disorders
Survey of all children aged 9–11 on the Isle of Wight (Rutter and Graham 1970)	42% (teacher reports) and 30% (parental reports) in those with IQ less than 70. Prevalence rate five times higher than control peers. Use of IQ alone to define learning disability is a major drawback
All youngsters aged 13 to 17 born in a Swedish urban area (Gillberg et al. 1986)	Psychiatric interviews based on DSM-III criteria; 64% with IQ less than 50 (severe learning disability) and 57% with IQ of 50 to 70 (mild learning disabilities) had a psychiatric disorder. Psychotic behaviour, conduct disorders, hyperactive disorder and emotional disorders common in mild learning disability. Use of IQ alone a drawback, but provided clear definitions of diagnostic criteria used
Representative sample of adults with learning disability from the Danish National Register using DSM-III criteria (Lund 1985)	Psychiatric diagnosis made in 27.1% ($n = 302$) of sample. Behaviour disorder (10%), dementia (22.2% in over-65s), schizophrenia (1.3%), affective disorder (1.7%) and psychosis of uncertain type (5%). Higher rate in those with active epilepsy

122 people with learning disability from the Swedish National Register. Psychiatric interviews based on DSM-III, Eysenck Personality Inventory and Comprehensive Psychopathology Rating Scale (1978) (Gostason 1985)	71% of severe learning disability, 33% of mild learning disability and 23% of control group received one or more psychiatric diagnoses
Community study, stratified random sampling, using the Psychopathology Instrument for Mentally Retarded Adults (PIMRA) (Iverson and Fox 1989)	Overall prevalence 35.9%; 54.5% in those with mild learning disability compared with 31.5% in moderate learning disability and 25.9% in severe learning disability.
Community study using a two-step methodology. Used Reiss Screen for Maladaptive Behaviour and further evaluation by psychologists (Reiss 1990)	Overall prevalence 39%; high rates for personality disorder (10.2%). Only 11.7% of participants had a psychiatric diagnosis recorded in their case notes, suggesting that mental disorder was underdiagnosed in this sample
Older people with moderate and severe learning disability. Used Psychiatric Assessment Schedule for Adults with a Developmental Disability (PAS-ADD) (Patel et al. 1993)	Overall prevalence 11.4%. Depression and anxiety were common. Prevalence of dementia was 11.4%. Used clearly defined criteria (ICD-9) and a structured and computerised method for obtaining a diagnosis
Prevalence study in Oxfordshire, 190 people with learning disability screened using Reiss Screen for Maladaptive Behaviour (Raghavan 2000)	67 people (35.2%) tested positive for mental disorder. More people tested positive in the moderate (23%) than in the mild (13.8%) learning disability category
Multicentre study in New South Wales, Australia. Used Developmental Behaviour Checklists and IQ (Enfield and Tonge 1996a and b)	40.7% of those aged 4 to 18 with learning disability classified as having severe emotional and behaviour disorders. Those with profound learning disability had lower levels of disturbance than those with mild, moderate and severe learning disability. Disruptive and antisocial behaviours more prominent in mild learning disability and 'self-absorbed' or 'autistic' behaviours more prominent in severe learning disability

Studies based on referred samples

The studies based on referred samples to psychiatrists also tend to show a higher prevalence estimate, with the exception of the Eaton and Menolascino study. People referred for psychiatric or psychological evaluation may be showing severe behaviour problems or confused mental states, and as a result this will lead to inflated prevalence estimates.

Study	Prevalence of psychiatric disorder
Those referred for psychiatric evaluation in Nebraska, USA (Eaton and Menolascino 1982)	14.3% of 798 people assessed had mental disorder using DSM-III criteria. 21% schizophrenia, 21% adjustment reaction, 29.8% organic brain syndrome with transient psychotic or behavioural reactions and 27.1% personality disorder
Adolescents referred for psychiatric evaluation (Myers 1987)	Most common diagnosis was conduct disorder (38.9%) using DSM-III criteria
Adults referred for psychiatric evaluation. In addition to psychiatric interview, used a range of measures such as Behaviour Problem Rating Scale and Clinical Psychopathology Mental Handicap Rating Scale (Bouras and Drummond 1992)	Prevalence 41% based on DSM-III-R criteria for people with expressive language. Schizophrenia/paranoid disorder 12.3%. Behaviour problems present in 52.5%

Studies based on hospital population

The prevalence studies based on hospital populations tend to underrepresent the population of people with learning disabilities because of referral biases and other selective factors (Rutter 1989). Hence, this could result in the inclusion of a misleadingly high proportion of subjects with multiple diagnoses. Naturally, the hospital population would contain a high percentage of people with mental health disorder and challenging behaviour, hence the high prevalence rate in these studies.

Study	Prevalence of psychiatric disorder
357 long-stay hospital residents aged 40 years and over (Day 1985)	30% had significant psychiatric disorder. 50.5% behaviour disorder, 27.5% psychoses, 9.2% organic disorders consisting of dementia and confused states, 3.7% anxiety disorders
Random sample of 100 people with learning disability in hospital (Ballinger et al. 1991)	ICD-9 diagnosis made in 80% of sample. High prevalence of psychoses and personality disorders
Large state residential facility in USA (Crews et al. 1994)	Total prevalence 5.5%. 8.87% had an affective disorder. Prevalence rate in this study lower than other hospital in-patient studies

Given the problems of appropriate diagnosis of mental health disorder, it is not surprising to observe a wide range of prevalence figures with little agreement among them. Estimates tend to vary from 15 to 80%, depending on the orientation and design of the study. The studies based on representative samples of the population indicate a prevalence of 30 to 40% and most of the policy documents and research papers tend to estimate the prevalence of mental illness in people with learning disability at 40%. A thorough review of most of the prevalence studies conducted until 1994 by Borthwick-Duffy (1994) concluded that a number of factors have influenced the prevalence figures. These include different definitions of what actually constitutes learning disabilities, dissimilarities in the population in each study and difference in research methodologies leading to different results. The inclusion of challenging behaviour in the diagnosis of mental health disorder and the use of a range of terms such as mental illness, mental disorder, psychiatric disorder, emotional disorder and behavioural disorder hinder the accurate detection, diagnosis and estimation of prevalence.

The use of various labels often reflects the psychological and theoretical background of people with learning disabilities, which often distorts the objective diagnosis (Szymanski 1980). The incidence of challenging behaviours or behaviour problems often overlaps with mental health disorder, which accounts for major confusion among clinicians and untrained carers alike in the process of detection and diagnosis. Hence, this is explored in the next section in order to throw more light on the intricacies of the overlap between behaviour and mental health disorders.

Challenging behaviour and mental health disorders

People with learning disabilities show severe behaviour problems or challenging behaviours, which pose a serious problem to health care services (Emerson et al. 1988; Emerson 1995). Challenging behaviour is defined as:

> 'behaviour of such an intensity, frequency or duration that the physical safety of the person or others is likely to be placed in serious jeopardy, or behaviour that is likely to seriously limit or deny access to the use of ordinary community services.' (Emerson et al. 1988, p. 16)

The term challenging behaviour covers a wide spectrum of behaviours, such as aggression, self-injurious behaviour, destruction of property, sexually inappropriate behaviour and eccentric habits, to mention a few (see Emerson et al. 1987 for comprehensive details on challenging behaviour). The extent of overlap between challenging behaviour and mental health disorder has been the subject of much debate and its impact on the detection and diagnosis of mental health disorders in people with learning disabilities is very confusing. People with challenging behaviour represent one of the largest groups who are referred to psychiatric or psychology services (Moss et al. 1997). Differential diagnosis of challenging behaviour and mental health disorder may have serious consequences on the understanding of the therapeutic needs of this population. For example, violent behaviour sometimes apparent in paranoid schizophrenia and social withdrawal accompanying clinical depression can be described as challenging behaviour.

The terminology that professionals use in the assessment and treatment of mental health disorder has added much confusion to the overlap between mental health disorder and challenging behaviour. Often professionals use 'behaviour disturbance' and 'psychiatric illness' interchangeably in regard to people with learning disabilities (Russel and Tanguay 1981). In their study of psychiatric and behaviour disturbance in people with learning disabilities, Fraser et al. (1986) suggested that behaviour disturbances in general are not expressions of psychiatric disturbances, according to their observation of clinical features in a psychiatric interview.

It has been suggested that challenging or disturbed behaviours are those that create problems in the interaction, care and management of people with learning disabilities, and hence Fraser et al. (1986) clearly oppose the use of the terms 'behaviour disturbance' and 'psychiatric disorder' interchangeably. It is argued that for some people behaviour problems or challenging behaviour may reflect the individual's interpersonal skill development without underlying psychopathology, but in other cases the same behavioural difficulties and stunted social development may be found as being symptomatic of an underlying mental health disorder (Dosen 1993). The case study below highlights challenging behaviour in mental illness.

Pat is 34 years old and lives in a group home, which she shares with two other clients. Pat has moderate learning disabilities, Prader–Willi syndrome and challenging behaviour. Her behavioural problems consist of both verbal and physical aggression to the extent that her placement is at risk. She has been progressively deteriorating in this regard over the past six months. She shares a house with one other resident whom she tries to dominate in all activities. Her carers have found it increasingly difficult to cope with her difficult behaviour. Staff have noticed that Pat has become much more irritable, with frequent temper outbursts mainly consisting of verbal abuse to others. She seems to be excessively tired all day and when angry is very difficult to reason with or support. She has become more rebellious. She has had recent medical problems with a fistula between her large intestine and bladder, which has resulted in pain and repeated infections. In view of the increased frequency and severity of her aggression, which is evident both at home and in public, there is a risk of her placement breaking down.

The overlap of challenging behaviour and mental health disorders has been examined from different perspectives. Moss et al. (2000) conducted a study to determine the proportion of people with challenging behaviour who have additional psychiatric symptoms. They surveyed 320 people with learning disabilities, with and without challenging behaviour, checking for the presence of psychiatric symptoms using the Psychiatric Assessment Schedule for Adults with a Developmental Disability (PAS-ADD) (Moss et al. 1998). Their study indicated that the increasing severity of challenging behaviour is associated with increased prevalence of psychiatric symptoms. An important finding from this study is that depression was four times more prevalent in people with challenging behaviour. Moss et al. suggest that the strong association with depression is significant because this condition is often undetected in the general population and in people with learning disabilities. Based on this association, they highlight that there may be many people with learning disabilities and challenging behaviour who may also have unrecognised psychiatric symptoms.

The prescription of psychotropic medication for challenging behaviour is another area of serious concern (Rodgers and Russell 1995) as it contributes to the clouding of the overlap between challenging behaviour and mental health disorder. There is evidence from the literature (Enfield 1992) that such medication may have been overprescribed on inadequate indications, and without proper analysis of the nature and function of challenging behaviour. Hubert (1992), in an in-depth study of 20 young adults classified as having severe learning disabilities and challenging behaviour living at home with their families, found that many young people were prescribed one or more antipsychotic drugs over many years without a diagnosis of mental health disorder.

Some tentative links have also been established between challenging behaviour and mental health disorders. In a study of depression in people with learning disabilities, Sovner and DesNoyers-Hurley (1983) suggested that depressive affect and cognition were often indirectly expressed, with aggressive acting out, withdrawal and somatic complaints occurring more commonly. Similarly, Reiss and Rojahn (1993) studied the relationship between aggression and depression, which led to their observation that the presence of depression was associated with a four-fold increase in the probability of an aggressive behaviour problem. A case report by Lowery and Sovner (1992) shows the relationship between aggression or self-injurious behaviour (SIB) and one phase of rapid cycling bipolar disorder. The link between challenging behaviour and mood disorders has been explored by Lowery (1993). He suggests that among the 48 published case reports of mood disorders examined, 11 people also exhibited aggressive behaviour, four displayed SIB and two had both aggression and SIB. He explored these further, and found that aggression co-existed with depressive episodes in three cases, while SIB and depression occurred in three other individuals. In relation to mania and challenging behaviour, Lowery reported 11 individuals who simultaneously displayed manic episodes and aggression and four who exhibited SIB and mania. He found that 35% of individuals with learning disabilities and mood disorder also displayed aggression or SIB. However, as this is based on a compilation of published case reports, this should not be treated as a prevalence figure. The study by Meins (1993) further explored symptoms connected with depression and found that aggressive and SIB stereotypes, screaming and spontaneous crying may be associated with depression in people with severe learning disabilities.

Thus the complex nature of this overlap should be taken into account when diagnosing mental health disorders in people with learning disabilities. Dosen (1993) argues that the area of overlap is broad and that this should not be a reason to abandon efforts to distinguish between challenging behaviour and mental health disorders. Hence, multidisciplinary assessment may be the best option for establishing appropriate diagnosis and treatment.

Prevalence – types of mental disorders

In the first part of this chapter we examined the prevalence studies and the overall prevalence estimates of mental health disorders in people with learning disabilities. In this section we focus on specific mental health disorders such as anxiety, depression, schizophrenia, dementia and personality disorders and the prevalence of these disorders in people with learning disabilities.

Prevalence of anxiety disorder

The prevalence rate of anxiety disorders varies significantly for the different subtypes of anxiety disorders, so that some subtypes are less common in people with a learning disability and others are more common or as common as those in the general population (Reiss 1993). Several studies have examined the occurrence of anxiety disorders in people with a learning disability living in hospital and community settings.

Phillips and Williams (1975), in their study of 100 outpatients, did not report anxiety disorders separately, but noted that anxiety reactions frequently accompanied another diagnosis. In their comprehensive survey of an English community, Richardson et al. (1979) found that 26% of young adults with a learning disability were thought to have experienced neurotic disorders. Reid (1980) found that 22% of 60 children who attended an outpatient clinic had neurotic diagnosis. In a survey of 130 children and adults attending an outpatient mental health clinic, 25% were diagnosed as either conduct or anxious-withdrawal disorders (Benson 1985). In a study covering a 5-year period of admissions to a hospital for mental health treatment, Day (1985) found that 28% of admissions were diagnosed as neurotic.

Bouras and Drummond (1992) identified that 6.6% of community residents referred to a mental health clinic for people with learning disability had a diagnosis of anxiety disorder using DSM-III criteria. In a prevalence study of psychiatric disorders in older people with a learning disability, Patel et al. (1993) found that 5.7% showed anxiety disorders.

The following story of Mark highlights the case of a person with learning disabilities living in residential accommodation.

Mark is a 29-year-old man with mild learning disabilities who lives in a home with one other resident. He has been in his present home for 10 years. Mark is described as having always been an anxious person, is very sociable and likes to keep himself busy. He has good independent living skills. He is able to use public transport independently once he knows the bus routes, he regularly goes to football matches, and is very competent shopping at supermarkets. He goes to a local college. He also works 3 days a week at a local shop. Mark has had a girlfriend for the past 2 years, but it seems that at times this relationship is stressful for him. Mark has perfectionist traits in his personality and likes to do things in a set routine. He gets quite anxious and restless when his routine is disrupted.

His carers report that Mark is becoming more anxious and insecure, which is associated with periodic irritability, reduced humour and a sad facial expression. His sleep pattern fluctuates, as does his appetite. He does not appear to be unduly tired. However, he does seem to be more restless and is finding it difficult to relax. He likes to keep busy and thus tends to be 'on the go' all the time. He likes to please others and thus cannot say no when asked to do tasks. Thus he ends up doing things that he may not necessarily want to do, resulting in bouts of irritability. He is suggestible and passive and appears to lack self-confidence. Mark continues to have an active social life and enjoys a number of different leisure pursuits. He denies feeling low in his mood and continues to be optimistic about the future.

McNally and Ascher (1987) highlighted the lack of data on the prevalence of panic disorder or agoraphobia in people with learning disability. However, Craft (1960) reported that 10.8% of learning disabled outpatients suffered from an 'anxiety state', which may indicate that this population is not immune to panic attacks. Chamblass (1985) argued and shattered the myth that agoraphobia occurs mostly in those who are highly intelligent and imaginative. This is based on the finding that at least some of the agoraphobics may be functioning in the borderline to mild classification of learning disability.

Certain unusual behaviours in people with a learning disability might actually be compulsive behaviours (Gedye 1992). There are problems in differentiating obsessive–compulsive behaviours (OCD) from stereotypic behaviours, which are most common in people with a learning disability. Vitiello et al. (1989) suggested that the compulsive behaviours that were found in their sample of people with a learning disability were reliably diagnosed and differentiated from stereotypes and other repetitive behaviours. This supports a concept of OCD based on external observation of repetitive, ritualistic behaviour and of its functional consequences. However, Reid (1985) believes that it requires a degree of intellectual sophistication to experience and describe the various components of true obsessional symptomatology, including the feeling of subjective compulsion, the struggle against compulsion and the retention of insight. Hence, Reid argues that people with a severe learning disability may not experience obsessive neurosis and he holds the view that some deeply engrained rituals and stereotypic behaviours should not be confused with obsessions.

There is also evidence from the literature to suggest that people with a learning disability are exposed to trauma and abuse more frequently than the general population (Sobsey 1994; Ryan 1995). Characteristics of post-traumatic stress disorder (PTSD) include the re-experiencing of the trauma in the form of intrusive thoughts, flashbacks and nightmares. It is also reported that people with a learning disability may be particularly susceptible to emotional problems such as PTSD following the death of a parent (Ollendick and Ollendick 1982).

The notion of low intelligence of this client group may suggest that the expression of PTSD may be low, but there is no reason to believe that these people are immune to the effects of stress reactions following physical and sexual abuse, traffic accidents and death of a relative. With the move towards ordinary living, as much as it might be in the best interests of the person for increasing the opportunities for quality life, the stress of relocation from a familiar environment and friends to a strange one may cause trauma (Heller 1984).

Prevalence of affective disorder

It is currently estimated that depressive episodes in adults with learning disabilities have a point prevalence of about 4% (Smiley and Cooper 2003). There have been no large-scale population-based epidemiological studies using standardised diagnostic criteria in adults with learning disabilities to give us more accurate information.

Studies by Reid (1976) and Carlson (1979) have established that people with a learning disability suffer from the full range of affective disorders experienced by the rest of the population. It is believed that people with a learning disability may actually have an increased vulnerability to affective disorders with earlier age of onset when compared to the general population (Reid 1985). Several hospital surveys report a prevalence rate of around 1.5% for service users suffering from an episode of affective psychosis (Reid 1985). Wright (1982) found a prevalence rate of 2.8% of affective disorders among 1507 people with a learning disability living in an institution, with the rate rising to 5.5% when atypical forms of affective disorders were included. Reiss (1993) reports a prevalence rate of 3 to 6% for affective disorders in the general population of people with a learning disability.

Glue (1989), in a study of a group of ten hospitalised people with learning disabilities with rapid cycling affective disorder, found that men had an earlier onset of affective illness and more rapid cycling than women. However, larger studies carried out in the general population have failed to report this pattern (Wher et al. 1988). Lowery and Sovner (1992), in their discussion of two case reports of rapid cycling bipolar disorder with two adults with a learning disability, suggest a correlation with SIB.

Gardner (1967) reported four epidemiological studies in which depression of people with a learning disability is mentioned, but this lacks any definitive data due to study design weakness. In a survey of psychiatric disorders in a hospitalised population ($n = 314$), Craft (1959) reported only one case of depressive illness. Heaton-Ward (1977) reviewed individuals suspected of mental health disorder referred to him from three hospitals. He reported retrospective diagnosis for eight men and eight women as having recurring episodes of depression with or without mania from examination of medical and nursing notes.

In a study of adults with learning disabilities who were resident in a hospital, Reid (1972) identified 21 individuals with manic-depressive illness. Corbett (1979) studied all the children and adults with a learning disability ($n = 400$) who were in contact with health care services living in Camberwell. He found a history of depression or manic depression in 2% of the participants, whilst 2% were found to be depressed at the time of the study. Corbett concluded from his sample that depression was more common in people with mild rather than severe levels of learning disability.

Case reports of Angst et al. (1990) and Clarke and MacLeod (1993) suggest that people with mild learning disability experience recurrent brief depression. Recurrent brief depression is different from the depressive illness familiar to general practitioners (GPs) and psychiatrists in that the episodes of depression are both frequent and of shorter duration than usual.

Szymanski and Biederman (1984) suggest that the misconception that people with a learning disability in general and those with Down's syndrome in particular do not suffer from depressive disorders is an important roadblock preventing mental health professionals from recognising this disorder in this population. They report three case studies of two men and one woman with Down's syndrome suspected of having depression and anorexia nervosa. Depression has been found to be three times more likely to occur in people with Down's syndrome than in people with learning disability of other aetiologies (Callacott et al. 1992). However, Meins (1993) asserts that there is no sign of any heightened vulnerability to major depression in adults with Down's syndrome, based on his studies of prevalence and risk factors in adults with learning disability.

Prevalence of schizophrenia

As in the prevalence of other types of mental health disorders in this population, the prevalence of schizophrenia is also drawn from a number of studies. Corbett (1979) conducted a community survey in south London using data from the Camberwell Register. This study showed a prevalence of schizophrenia of 3% and this is comparable to the studies of Reid (1972) and Heaton-Ward (1977). The Swedish survey by Gostason (1985) identified four schizophrenic patients among 131 individuals as having severe or mild learning disability, which amounts to 3%. However, Gostason was reluctant to conclude this, due to the small sample considered in his study.

Lund (1985) in a Danish study using a normative sample and adopting criteria from DSM-III found an overall prevalence of 1.3% for schizophrenia. However, rates of 3.3% for those in the IQ range 85 to 68 and 2.6% for those in the IQ range 67 to 52 reflect the figures from other studies. Eaton and Menolascino (1982) in their study of people in a community-based programme in Nebraska referred for psychiatric assessment using DSM-III criteria found that 21% of the sample were diagnosed as having schizophrenia.

Hospital studies show a higher prevalence in this population (Hucker et al. 1979; Russel and Tanguay 1981). Like other illnesses, the detection and diagnosis of schizophrenia greatly depend on the characteristics of the population studied and hence hospital studies show a higher prevalence as opposed to community surveys. Most studies have reported rates of schizophrenia in people with learning disabilities to be about 3%. This compares with estimates of 0.6 to 3% for the general population. Recently there has been an upsurge in the number of case reports connecting learning disability, schizophrenia and Down's syndrome (Cooper and Callacott 1994, 1996; Duggirala et al. 1995).

It is believed that the age and onset of schizophrenia in people with learning disabilities are similar to those in the ordinary 'normal' population. However, there is a lack of scientific studies to arrive at this conclusion (Turner 1989). There is also no proven association between physical pathology and schizophrenia in people with learning disability (Reid 1985). However, as schizophrenia occurs in people with a wide range of neurological disabilities including epilepsy, it is not clear whether epilepsy and schizophrenia in this population are causal or coincidental.

Prevalence of dementia

The extent to which individuals with learning disabilities and other developmental disorders are at increased risk of developing dementia associated with Alzheimer's disease is not clear (Zigman et al. 1995). Various estimates of the prevalence of dementia in people with learning disabilities are given in the literature. Burt et al. (1995) in a cross-sectional study of 61 people with learning disabilities (aged 20 to 60) found a prevalence of 8.2%. An autopsy study by Cole et al. (1994) of 12 people with learning disability and Down's syndrome (age range 36 to 65 years) identified a prevalence of 83.3%.

The prevalence study of dementia in people with Down's syndrome by Prasher (1995) is based on population prevalence. The prevalence study of dementia in people with learning disability from all causes by Cooper (1997) is based on a sample of adults with learning disabilities in community settings. Hoffman et al. (1991) compared these prevalence estimates with a European prevalence study of dementia in the general population. As indicated in Table 3.1, the prevalence of dementia is higher in people with Down's syndrome than in people with learning disabilities from all causes and the general population.

Prevalence of personality disorder

Only a few reports identify the prevalence of personality disorder in people with learning disability. Eaton and Menolascino (1982) found that 27% of a sample of 115 people with learning disability and mental illness in a community programme were additionally diagnosed with a personality disorder and

Table 3.1 Prevalence of dementia in people with Down's syndrome, with learning disability and in the general population.

Down's syndrome		Learning disability (all causes)		General population	
Age range	Incidence (%)	Age range	Incidence (%)	Age range	Incidence (%)
30–39	2.0	65–74	15.6	60–64	1.0
40–49	9.4	75–84	23.5	65–69	1.4
50–59	36.1	85–94	70.0	70–74	4.1
60–69	54.5			75–79	5.7
				80–84	13.0
				85–89	21.6
				90–95	32.2

Adapted from Hoffman et al. (1991), Prasher (1995) and Cooper (1997).

suggest that antisocial personality is the most frequently diagnosed form of personality disorder. Ballinger and Reid (1987), in their study of 100 mild and moderate in-patients with learning disability using the Standardised Assessment of Personality (Mann et al. 1981), found personality abnormalities in 56% of the population, of which 22% had severe abnormalities indicating a personality disorder. Deb and Hunter (1991) suggest that the prevalence of personality disorder in people with learning disabilities living in community settings is lower than those in hospital settings. This is based on their assertion that the presence of personality disorder is a 'major exclusion criterion' for the rehabilitation and integration of these people from hospital to community settings.

Causative factors

Very little is known about the causes of mental illness in people with learning disabilities. In the absence of substantive research data on identifiable causes of the high prevalence of mental illness in this population, we are compelled to rely on tentative links identified in some studies and assumptions based on the general population. Hence, the possible causative factors for the development of mental illness in people with learning disabilities require further in-depth examination.

Matson and Sevin (1994) in their paper outlining the theories of dual diagnosis highlight a number of links to biological, psychological and social causative factors. To this we have added other identifiable links that have been published since the Matson and Sevin paper.

Key biological factors

The biological factors that may predispose a person with learning disabilities to develop mental illness are as follows:

- Structural brain pathologies (Matson and Sevin 1994).
- Psychiatric disorders are more common in children with learning disabilities with neurological abnormalities than in children without these abnormalities (Rutter 1971).
- Head trauma and other neurological conditions are associated with increased prevalence of emotional disorders in children with learning disabilities (Rutter 1981; Gostason 1985).
- Development of Alzheimer's-related dementia and associated depression in people with Down's syndrome (Matson and Sevin 1994; Oliver and Holland 1986).
- Reports of high prevalence of anxiety disorders in people with learning disabilities with fragile X syndrome (Bregman et al. 1988).
- There is a link between epilepsy and increased prevalence of psychopathology in people with learning disabilities (Rutter et al. 1970; Lund 1985; Reid 1985).
- The high prevalence of emotional disorders in people with hearing and visual impairments and learning disabilities (Rutter et al. 1970).
- The side effects of medications and associated problems (Tyrer and Hill 2001).

Key psychological factors

- Transition into adulthood and the related psychological and social impacts on the individual and the family (Masi 1998; McIntyre et al. 2002).
- Abnormal developmental processes in children with a learning disability – fragile emotional attachments, slower development of self and object constancy, impaired symbol formation and separation–individuation from the parent are significantly affected (Levitas and Gilson 1990; Gaedt 2003; Whittaker 2001).
- Acquiring fears and phobia as a result of observation or modelling of other individuals suffering anxiety towards an object or event (Matson and Sevin 1994). This connects to the social learning model of learning maladaptive behaviours.
- Limited opportunities for the learning and fostering of appropriate behaviour, new skills and abilities in the living environment.
- Lack of appropriate support and encouragement for children with learning disabilities at school (Weisz 1990).
- Isolation, social skills deficit, social anxiety and depression (Reiss and Benson 1985; Helsel and Matson 1988; Matson et al. 2000).
- Limited intellectual capacity for solving problems and limited ability to adopt appropriate and effective coping mechanisms.
- The lifelong dependency upon others and the demands of society upon individuals with a learning disability as they grow up can further burden already fragile psychological defences (Menolascino 1990).
- Life experiences which lead to learned deficits in motivation, feelings of worthlessness and other symptoms of depression (Matson and Sevin 1994).

- People with learning disabilities with physical deformities – low self-esteem and problems with interaction (Bijou 1966).
- Uncertainty and fear of failure (Dosen 1984) and learned helplessness (Weisz 1990). Higher expectancies of failure and the attribution of failure to internal factors may increase levels of anxiety (Matson and Sevin 1994).
- Psychopathological behaviours may be maintained through positive reinforcement (Matson and Sevin 1994).
- Individuals with learning disabilities are more vulnerable than others to becoming victims of abuse (Sinason 1992).
- The relationship between depression and self-injurious behaviour (Lowery and Sovner 1992; Marston et al. 1997; Ross and Oliver 2002).

Key social factors

- Exposure to negative social experiences – segregation from ordinary social experiences due to restrictive placements or carers seeking to protect the individual from possible stigma and ridicule (Matson and Sevin 1994).
- Isolation and limited opportunities for socialisation in group homes may contribute to depression (Matson and Sevin 1994).
- Restricted access to employment, social prejudices and continued dependency on others (Reiss and Benson 1984).
- Labelling, stigma and low self-esteem and prolonged exposure to negative social conditions (Reiss and Benson 1984).
- Encountering more difficulties in ordinary day-to-day living, while having a reduced capacity to handle these problems (Matson and Sevin 1994).
- Families supporting children with learning disabilities are more likely to be subject to social and material disadvantages compared to families supporting children with no learning disabilities (Emerson 2003).
- There is a high prevalence of mental illness in young people with learning disabilities, owing to associations with social disadvantage (lower social class and reduced household income), being cared for by a lone parent, 'unhealthy' patterns of family functioning, punitive child management practices and carer mental distress (Emerson 2003).
- Discrimination on the grounds of race, gender, culture or sexual orientation. The burden of care in South Asian families is greater than that in white families both socially and financially, compounded by severe problems of poverty, bad housing, racism and higher levels of unemployment (Butt and Mizra 1996).

Understanding the nature and manifestation of dual diagnosis

As we have seen, the nature and manifestation of mental illness in people with learning disabilities is a complex and confusing process. Nurses and other care staff working with people with learning disabilities need to take account of the following in order to help them have a better understanding of the nature and manifestation of dual diagnosis:

- A good understanding of the level of functioning of the person through assessment of skills, abilities and emotional states and behaviours.
- Screening for mental illness and in-depth exploration or investigation of the physical and mental states of the person.
- Record-keeping of the assessment and care plans. Providing a descriptive account of the implementation of care plans, paying special attention to emotional and behavioural variations on a day-to-day basis.
- Exploration of culturally inappropriate behaviours through functional analysis, understanding the triggers and maintaining factors.
- Being knowledgeable and competent: exploring and identifying the key issues of the person and seeking appropriate professional advice and help; guiding junior nurses and frontline staff in the assessment process; supervising the implementation of assessments and intervention or care plans; evaluating their impact on the person's daily living and activities.

The complex nature of dual diagnosis presents a range of therapeutic challenges, which requires distinct responses from clinical practitioners and service providers.

Conclusion

The discussion of the nature, causes and prevalence of various mental health disorders among people with learning disabilities has highlighted the spectrum of mental health disorders normally experienced by young people, adults and older people with learning disabilities. The literature clearly indicates a high prevalence of mental health disorders in this population, despite some of the methodological weaknesses of these studies. For example, most of the studies failed to define learning disabilities and lack information relating to the inclusion criteria. The range and types of diagnostic methods used also indicate confusion in this area due to the various adaptations to the diagnostic procedure by clinicians and researchers. In addition to these factors, the population studied fall under various criteria such as hospital populations, referral to psychiatrists and random samples. However, it is safe to estimate an overall prevalence rate of 27 to 40% based on studies conducted with representative samples.

References

Angst, J., Merikangas, K., Scheidegger, P. and Wicki, W. (1990) Recurrent brief depression: a new subtype of affective disorder. *Journal of Affective Disorders*, **19**, 87–98.

Ballinger, B.R. and Reid, A.H. (1987) A standardised assessment of personality disorder in mental handicap. *British Journal of Psychiatry*, **150**, 108–109.

Ballinger, B.R., Ballinger, C.B., Reid, A.H. and McQueen, E. (1991) The psychiatric symptoms, diagnoses and care needs of 100 mentally handicapped patients. *British Journal of Psychiatry*, **158**, 255–259.

Benson, B.A. (1985) Behaviour disorders and mental retardation: association with age, sex and level of functioning in an outpatient clinic sample. *Applied Research in Mental Retardation*, **6**, 79–85.

Bijou, S.W. (1966) A functional analysis of retarded development. In: N.R. Ellis (Ed.) *International Review of Research in Mental Retardation*, Vol 1. San Diego: Academic Press.

Borthwick-Duffy, S.A. (1994) Epidemiology and prevalence of psychopathology in people with mental retardation. *Journal of Consulting and Clinical Psychology*, **62**, 17–27.

Bouras, N. and Drummond, C. (1992) Behaviour and psychiatric disorders of people with mental handicaps living in the community. *Journal of Intellectual Disability Research*, **36**, 349–357.

Bregman, J.D., Leckman, J.F. and Ort, S.I. (1988) Fragile X syndrome: genetic predisposition to psychopathology. *Journal of Autism and Developmental Disorders*, **18**, 343–354.

Burt, D.B., Loveland, K.A., Chen, Y.W., Chuang, A., Lewis, K.R. and Cherry, L. (1995) Ageing in adults with Down's syndrome: report from a longitudinal study. *American Journal on Mental Retardation*, **100**, 262–270.

Butt, J. and Mizra, K. (1996) *Social Care and Black Communities*. London: HMSO.

Callacott, R.A., Cooper, S.A. and McGrother, C. (1992) Differential rates of psychiatric disorders in adults with Down's syndrome compared with other mentally handicapped adults. *British Journal of Psychiatry*, **161**, 671–674.

Carlson, G. (1979) Affective psychoses in mental retardates. *Psychiatry Clinical North America*, **2**, 499–510.

Chamblass, D.L. (1985) The relationship of severity agoraphobia to associated psychopathology. *Behaviour Research and Therapy*, **23**, 305–310.

Clarke, D.J. and MacLeod, M. (1993) Recurrent brief depression and mild learning disability: successful community management. *Mental Handicap*, **21**, 92–96.

Cole, G., Neal, J.W., Fraser, W.I. and Cowie, V.A. (1994) Autopsy findings in patients with mental handicap. *Journal of Intellectual Disability Research*, **38**, 9–26.

Cooper, S.A. (1997) High prevalence of dementia amongst people with learning disabilities not attributed to Down's syndrome. *Irish Journal of Psychological Medicine*, **27**, 609–616.

Cooper, S.A. and Callacott, R. (1994) Clinical features and diagnostic criteria of depression in Down's syndrome. *British Journal of Psychiatry*, **165**, 399–403.

Cooper, S.A. and Callacott, R. (1996) Depressive episodes in adults with learning disabilities. *Irish Journal of Psychological Medicine*, **13**, 105–113.

Corbett, J.A. (1979) Psychiatric morbidity and mental retardation. In: F.E. James and R.P. Snaith (Eds) *Psychiatric Illness and Mental Handicap*. London: Gaskell.

Craft, M. (1959) Mental disorder in the defective: a psychiatric survey among in-patients. *American Journal of Mental Deficiency*, **64**, 829–834.

Craft, M. (1960) Mental disorder in a series of English outpatient defectives. *American Journal of Mental Deficiency*, **64**, 718–724.

Crews, D.W. Jr, Bonaventura, S. and Rowe, F. (1994) Dual diagnosis: prevalence of psychiatric disorders in a large state residential facility for individuals with mental retardation. *American Journal of Mental Retardation*, **98**, 688–731.

Day, K. (1985) Psychiatric disorders in the middle aged and elderly mentally handicapped. *British Journal of Psychiatry*, **147**, 660–667.

Deb, S. and Hunter, D. (1991) Psychopathology of people with mental handicap and epilepsy, III: personality disorder. *British Journal of Psychiatry*, **159**, 830–834.

Dosen, A. (1984) Depressive conditions in mentally handicapped children. *Acta Paedopsychiatricia*, **50**, 29–40.

Dosen, A. (1993) Mental health and mental illness in persons with retardation: what are we talking about? In: R. Fletcher and A. Dosen (Eds) *Mental Health Aspects of Mental Retardation*. New York: Lexington Books.

Duggirala, C., Cooper, S.A. and Callacott, R.A. (1995) Schizophrenia and Down's syndrome. *Irish Journal of Psychological Medicine*, **12**, 30–33.

Eaton, L.F. and Menolascino, F.J. (1982) Psychiatric disorders in the mentally retarded: types, problems and challenges. *American Journal of Psychiatry*, **139**, 1297–1303.

Emerson, E. (1995) *Challenging Behaviour: Analysis and Intervention in People with Learning Disabilities*. Cambridge: Cambridge University Press.

Emerson, E. (2003) Prevalence of psychiatric disorders in children and adolescents with and without intellectual disability. *Journal of Intellectual Disability Research*, **47**, 51–58.

Emerson, E., Toogood, A., Mansell, J. et al. (1988) Challenging behaviour and community services: 2. Who are the people who challenge services? *Mental Handicap*, **16**, 16–19.

Emerson, E., Toogood, A., Mansell, J. et al. (1987) Challenging behaviour and community services: 1. Introduction and overview. *Mental Handicap*, **15**, 166–169.

Enfield, S.L. (1992) Clinical assessment of psychiatric symptoms in mentally retarded individuals. *Australian and New Zealand Journal of Psychiatry*, **26**, 48–63.

Enfield, S.L. and Tonge, B.J. (1996a) Population prevalence of psychopathology in children and adolescents with intellectual disability: I. Rationale and methods. *Journal of Intellectual Disability Research*, **40**, 91–98.

Enfield, S.L. and Tonge, B.J. (1996b) Population prevalence of psychopathology in children and adolescents with intellectual disability: II. Epidemiological findings. *Journal of Intellectual Disability Research*, **40**, 99–109.

Fraser, W.I., Leuder, I., Gray, J. and Campbell, I. (1986) Psychiatric and behaviour disturbance in mental handicap. *Journal of Mental Deficiency Research*, **30**, 49–57.

Gaedt, C. (2003) Psychodynamically oriented psychotherapy in mentally retarded children. In: A. Dosen and K. Day (Eds) *Treating Mental Illness and Behaviour Disorders in Children and Adults with Mental Retardation*. Washington DC: American Psychiatric Press.

Gardner, W.I. (1967) Occurrence of severe depressive reactions in the mentally retarded. *American Journal of Psychiatry*, **124**, 386–388.

Gedye, A. (1992) Recognising obsessive–compulsive disorder claims in clients with developmental disabilities. *The Habilitative Mental Health Care Newsletter*, **11**, 73–74.

Gelder, M., Mayou, R. and Cowen, P. (2001) *Short Oxford Textbook of Psychiatry*. Oxford: Oxford Medical Illustrations.

Gillberg, C., Persson, E., Grufman, M. and Themner, U. (1986) Psychiatric disorders in mildly and severely mentally retarded urban children and adolescents: epidemiological aspects. *British Journal of Psychiatry*, **149**, 68–74.

Glue, P. (1989) Rapid cycling affective disorders in the mentally retarded. *Biological Psychiatry*, **26**, 250–256.

Gostason, R. (1985) Psychiatric illness among the mentally retarded. A Swedish population study. *Acta Psychiatrica Scandinavica*, **71** (Suppl. 318), 1–107.

Heaton-Ward, A. (1977) Psychosis in mental handicap. *British Journal of Psychiatry*, **130**, 525–533.

Heller, T. (1984) Issues in adjustment of mentally retarded individuals to residential relocation. *International Review of Research in Mental Retardation*, **12**, 123–147.

Helsel, W.J. and Matson, J.L. (1988) The relationship of depression to social skills and intellectual functioning in mentally retarded adults. *Journal of Mental Deficiency Research*, **32**, 411–418.

Hoffman, A., Rocca, W.A., Brayne, C. et al. (1991) The prevalence of dementia in Europe: a collaborative study of 1980–1990 findings. *International Journal of Epidemiology*, **20**, 736–748.

Hubert, J. (1992) *Too Many Drugs, Too Little Care, Parents' Perceptions of Administration and Side Effects of Drugs Prescribed for Young People with Severe Learning Difficulties*. London: Values Into Action.

Hucker, S.J., Day, K.A., George, S. and Roth, M. (1979) Psychosis in mentally retarded adults. In: F.E. James and R.P. Snaith (Eds) *Psychiatric Illness and Mental Handicap*. Special Publication of the Royal College of Psychiatrists. Ashford: Headley Brothers.

Iverson, J.C. and Fox, R.A. (1989) Prevalence of psychopathology among mentally retarded adults. *Research in Developmental Disabilities*, **10**, 77–83.

Levitas, A. and Gilson, S. (1990) *Towards the Developmental Understanding of the Impact of Mental Retardation on Assessment and Psychopathology*. Rockville, Maryland: National Institute for Mental Health.

Lowery, M.A. (1993) Behavioural psychology update: a clear link between problems, behaviours and mood disorders. *The Habilitative Mental Health Care Newsletter*, **12**, 105–110.

Lowery, M.A. and Sovner, R. (1992) Severe behaviour problems associated with rapid cycling bipolar disorder in two adults with profound mental retardation. *Journal of Intellectual Disability Research*, **36**, 269–281.

Lund, J. (1985) The prevalence of psychiatric morbidity in mentally retarded adults. *Acta Psychiatrica Scandinavica*, **72**, 563–570.

Mann, A.H., Jenkins, R., Cutting, J.C. and Cowen, P.J. (1981) The development and use of a standardised assessment of abnormal personality. *Psychological Medicine*, **11**, 839–847.

Marston, G.M., Perry, D.W. and Roy, A. (1997) Manifestation of depression in people with intellectual disability. *Journal of Intellectual Disability Research*, **41**, 476–480.

Masi, G. (1998) Psychiatric illness in mentally retarded adolescents: clinical features. *Adolescence*, **33**, 425–434.

Matson, J.L. and Sevin, J.A. (1994) Theories of dual diagnosis in mental retardation. *Journal of Consulting and Clinical Psychology*, **62**, 6–16.

Matson, J.L., Anderson, S.J. and Bamburg, J.W. (2000) The relationship of social skills to psychopathology for individuals with mild and moderate mental retardation. *British Journal of Developmental Disabilities*, **46**, 15–21.

McIntyre, L.L., Blacher, J. and Baker, B.L. (2002) Behaviour/mental health problems in young adults with intellectual disability: the impact on families. *Journal of Intellectual Disability Research*, **46**, 239–249.

McNally, R.J. and Ascher, L.M. (1987) Anxiety disorders in mentally retarded people. In: L. Michelson and L.M. Ascher (Eds) *Anxiety and Stress Disorders: Cognitive–Behavioural Assessment and Treatment*. New York: Guilford Press.

Meins, W. (1993) Prevalence and risk factors for depressive disorders in adults with intellectual disability. *Australia and New Zealand Journal of Developmental Disabilities*, **18**, 147–156.

Menolascino, F.J. (1990) Mental retardation and the risk, nature and types of mental illness. In: A. Dosen and F.J. Menolascino (Eds) *Depression in Mentally Retarded Children and Adults*. Leiden: Logon.

Moss, S., Emerson, E. and Kiernan, C. (2000) Psychiatric symptoms in adults with learning disabilities and challenging behaviour. *British Journal of Psychiatry*, **177**, 453–456.

Moss, S., Emerson, E., Bouras, N. and Holland, A. (1997) Mental disorders and problematic behaviours in people with intellectual disability: future directions for research. *Journal of Intellectual Disability Research*, **41**, 440–447.

Moss, S., Patel, P., Prosser, H. et al. (1993) Psychiatric morbidity in older people with moderate and severe learning disability. I: Development and reliability of the patient interview (PAS-ADD). *British Journal of Psychiatry*, **163**, 471–480.

Moss, S., Prosser, H., Costelleo, H., et al. (1998) Reliability and validity of the PAS-ADD checklist for detecting disorders in adults with intellectual disability. *Journal of Intellectual Disability Research*, **42** (2), 173–183.

Myres, B. (1987) Psychiatric problems in adolescents with developmental disabilities. *Journal of American Academy of Children and Adolescent Psychiatry*, **26**, 74–79.

Oliver, C. and Holland, A.J. (1986) Down's syndrome and Alzheimer's disease: a review. *Psychological Medicine*, **16**, 307–322.

Ollendick, T.H. and Ollendick, D.G. (1982) Anxiety disorders. In: J.L. Matson and R.P. Barrett (Eds) *Psychopathology in the Mentally Retarded*. New York: Grune and Stratton.

Patel, P., Goldberg, D. and Moss, S. (1993) Psychiatric morbidity in older people with moderate and severe learning disability: the prevalence study. *British Journal of Psychiatry*, **163**, 481–491.

Phillips, I. and Williams, N. (1975) Pathology and mental retardation: a study of 100 mentally retarded children: I. Psychopathology. *American Journal of Psychiatry*, **132**, 1265–1271.

Prasher, V.P. (1995) Age-specific prevalence, thyroid dysfunction and depressive symptomatology in adults with Down's syndrome and dementia. *International Journal of Geriatric Psychiatry*, **10**, 25–31.

Raghavan, R. (2000) An investigation into the needs of people with learning disabilities and mental health disorders (dual diagnosis). Thesis submitted to Oxford Brookes University.

Reid, A.H. (1972) Psychoses in adult mental defectives: I. Manic depressive psychosis. *British Journal of Psychiatry*, **120**, 205–212.

Reid, A.H. (1976) Psychiatric disturbances in the mentally handicapped. *Proceedings of the Royal Society of Medicine*, **69**, 509–512.

Reid, A.H. (1980) Psychiatric disorders in mentally handicapped children: a clinical and follow up study. *Journal of Mental Deficiency Research*, **24**, 287–298.

Reid, A.H. (1985) Psychiatry and mental handicap. In: M. Craft, J. Bicknell and S. Hollins (Eds) *Mental Handicap: A Multidisciplinary Approach*. East Sussex: Baillière Tindall.

Reiss, S. (1990) Prevalence of dual diagnosis in community-based day programs in the Chicago metropolitan area. *American Journal of Mental Retardation*, **94**, 578–585.

Reiss, S. (1993) Assessment of psychopathology in persons with mental retardation. In: J.L. Matson and R.P. Barrett (Eds) *Psychopathology in the Mentally Retarded*, 2nd Edition. Boston: Allyn and Bacan.

Reiss, S. and Benson, B. (1984) Awareness of negative social conditions among mentally retarded, emotionally disturbed outpatients. *American Journal of Psychiatry*, **141**, 88–90.

Reiss, S. and Benson, B. (1985) Psychosocial correlates of depression in mentally retarded adults: 1. Minimal social support and stigmatisation. *American Journal of Mental Deficiency*, **89**, 331–337.

Reiss, S. and Rojahn, J. (1993) Joint occurrence of depression and aggression in children and adults with mental retardation. *Journal of Intellectual Disability Research*, **37**, 287–294.

Richardson, S.A., Katz, M. and Koller, H. (1979) Some characteristics of a population of mentally retarded young adults in a British city: a basis for estimating some service needs. *Journal of Mental Deficiency Research*, **23**, 275–285.

Rodgers, J. and Russell, O. (1995) Healthy lives: the health needs of people with learning difficulties. In: T. Philpot and L. Ward (Eds) *Values and Visions: Changing Ideas for People with Learning Disabilities*. Oxford: Butterworth-Heinemann.

Ross, E. and Oliver, C. (2002) The relationship between levels of mood, interest and pleasure and 'challenging behaviour' in adults with severe and profound disability. *Journal of Intellectual Disability Research*, **46**, 191–197.

Russel, A.T. and Tanguay, P.E. (1981) Mental illness or mental retardation: cause or coincidence? *American Journal of Mental Deficiency*, **85**, 570–574.

Rutter, M. (1971) Psychiatry. In: J. Wortis (Ed.) *Mental Retardation: An Annual Review*, Vol 3. New York: Grune and Stratton.

Rutter, M. (1981) Psychological sequelae of brain damage in children. *American Journal of Psychiatry*, **138**, 1533–1544.

Rutter, M. (1989) Isle of Wight revisited: twenty-five years of children psychiatric epidemiology. *Journal of American Academy of Children and Adolescent Psychiatry*, **28**, 633–653.

Rutter, M. and Graham, P. (1970) Epidemiology of psychiatric disorder. In: M. Rutter., J. Tizard and K. Whitmore (Eds) *Education, Health, and Behaviour*. London: Longman Group.

Rutter, M., Tizard, J., Yule, W. and Graham, Y. (1970) *A Neuropsychiatric Study in Childhood Clinics in Developmental Medicine*, Nos 35/36. London: SIMP/Heinemann.

Ryan, R. (1995) Posttraumatic stress disorder in persons with developmental disabilities. *Community Mental Health Journal*, **30**, 45–54.

Sinason, V. (1992) *Mental Handicap and the Human Condition: New Approaches from the Tavistock*. London: Free Association Books.

Smiley, E. and Cooper, S.A. (2003) Intellectual disabilities, depressive episode, diagnostic criteria and diagnostic criteria for psychiatric disorders for use with adults with learning disabilities/mental retardation (DC-LD). *Journal of Intellectual Disability Research*, **47** (Suppl. 1), 62–71.

Sobsey, D. (1994) The research that shattered the myths: understanding the nature of abuse and abusers. *The National Association for the Dually Diagnosed (NADD) Newsletter*, **3**, 1–4.

Sovner, R. and DesNoyers-Hurley, A. (1983) Do the mentally retarded suffer from affective illness? *Archives of General Psychiatry*, **40**, 61–67.

Szymanski, L.S. (1980) Psychiatric diagnosis of retarded persons. In: L.S. Szymanski and P.E. Tanguay (Eds) *Emotional Disorders of Mentally Retarded Persons*. Baltimore: University Park Press.

Szymanski, L.S. and Biederman, J. (1984) Depression and anorexia nervosa of persons with Down's syndrome. *American Journal of Mental Deficiency*, **89**, 246–251.

Turner, T.H. (1989) Schizophrenia and mental handicap: an historical review, with implications for further research. *Psychological Medicine*, **19**, 301–314.

Tyrer, S. and Hill, S. (2001) Psychopharmacological approaches. In: A. Dosen and K. Day (Eds) *Treating Mental Illness and Behaviour Disorders in Children and Adults with Mental Retardation*. Washington DC: Psychiatric Press.

Vitiello, B., Spreat, S. and Behar, D. (1989) Obsessive–compulsive disorder in mentally retarded patients. *The Journal of Nervous and Mental Disease*, **177**, 232–236.

Weisz, J.R. (1990) Cultural–familial mental retardation: a developmental perspective on cognitive performance and 'helpless' behaviour. In: R.M. Hodapp, J.A. Burack and E. Zigler (Eds) *Issues in the Developmental Approach to Mental Retardation*. Cambridge: Cambridge University Press.

Wher, T.A., Sack, D.A., Rosenthal, N.E. and Cowdry, R.W. (1988) Rapid cycling affective disorder: contributing factors and treatment responses in 51 patients. *American Journal of Psychiatry*, **145**, 179–184.

Whittaker, S. (2001) Anger control for people with learning disabilities: a critical review. *Behavioural and Cognitive Psychotherapy*, **29**, 277–293.

World Health Organization (1993) *The ICD-10 Classification of Mental and Behavioural Disorders. Diagnostic Criteria for Research*. Geneva: WHO.

Wright, E.C. (1982) The presentation of mental illness in mentally retarded adults. *British Journal of Psychiatry*, **141**, 496–502.

Zigman, W.B., Schupf, N., Sersen, E. and Silverman, W. (1995) Prevalence of dementia in adults with and without Down's syndrome. *American Journal of Mental Retardation*, **100**, 403–412.

Further reading

Beadsmore, K., Dormamn, T., Cooper, S.-A. and Webb, T. (1998) Affective psychosis and Prader–Willi syndrome. *Journal of Intellectual Disability Research*, **42** (6), 463–471.

Clarke, D., Boer, H., Webb, T. et al. (1998) Prader–Willi syndrome and psychotic symptoms: 1. Case descriptions and genetic studies. *Journal of Intellectual Disability Research*, **42** (6), 440–450.

Clarke, D.J. (1993) Prader–Willi syndrome and psychoses. *British Journal of Psychiatry*, **163**, 680–684.

Cooke, L.B., Cooper, S.A. and Callacott, R.A. (1996) Depressive episodes in adults with learning disabilities. *Irish Journal of Psychological Medicine*, **13**, 105–113.

Deb, S. (1997) Behavioural phenotypes. In: S. Reed (Ed.) *Psychiatry in Learning Disabilities*. London: W.B. Saunders.

Dykens, E.M., Leckman, J.F. and Cassidy, S.B. (1996) Obsessions and compulsions in Prader–Willi syndrome. *Journal of Child Psychology and Psychiatry*, **37**, 995–1002.

Kollrack, H.W. and Wolff, D. (1966) Paranoid-halluzinatorische psychose bei Prader–Labhart–Willi–Fanconi syndrome. *Acta Paedopsychiatricia*, **33**, 309–314.

Navosal, S. (1984) Psychiatric disorder in adults admitted to a hospital for the mentally handicapped. *British Journal of Mental Subnormality*, **30**, 54–58.

Reiss, S. (1988) *The Reiss Screen for Maladaptive Behaviour*. Ohio: IDS Publishing.

Roy, A. and Cumella, S. (1993) Developing local services for people with a learning disability and psychiatric disorder. *Psychiatric Bulletin*, **17**, 215–217.

Sinason, V. (1998) Abuse of people with learning disabilities and other vulnerable adults. *Advances in Psychiatric Treatment*, **4**, 119–125.

Singh, N.N., Sood, A., Sonenklar, N. and Ellis, C. (1991) Assessment and diagnosis of mental illness in persons with mental retardation: methods and measures. *Behaviour Modification*, **15**, 419–443.

Verhoeven, W.M.A., Curfs, L.M.G. and Tuinier, S. (1998) Prader–Willi syndrome and cycloid psychoses. *Journal of Intellectual Disability Research*, **42** (6), 455–462.

Whittaker, J.F., Copper, C., Harrighton, R.C. and Price, D.A. (1977) Prader–Willi syndrome and acute psychosis. *International Journal of Psychiatry in Clinical Practice*, **1**, 217–219.

Chapter 4
Assessment and diagnosis

The detection and diagnosis of mental health disorders in people with learning disabilities is a complex process. There appears to be a general consensus amongst experts that the presentation of mental disorder in adults with borderline to mild learning disabilities is broadly similar in form to the way mental disorders present in the general population. However, the description of the individual symptoms may be less detailed and less reliable, and thus corroboration with information from others who know the person well becomes more important. In contrast the diagnosis of psychiatric disorders in those with severe and profound learning disabilities with poor communication presents more difficulties. In this group in particular the disorder is more likely to manifest as behavioural changes or changes in mood and biological functions, for example sleep, appetite, libido and energy levels. The applicability of diagnostic criteria derived from the general population to this group is particularly problematic, especially for disorders such as schizophrenia which rely on clear descriptions of bizarre and distressing mental phenomena.

Key themes

- Issues concerning and problems in the detection and diagnosis of mental health disorders in people with learning disabilities
- The use of diagnostic criteria for the assessment of mental health disorders
- The phenomenon of diagnostic overshadowing
- Manifestation of symptoms in people with learning disabilities
- Multiple diagnostic presentations and differential diagnosis
- Assessment in routine clinical practice
- Nursing contribution to assessment

Introduction

Assessment procedures are generally used to classify individuals into diagnostic categories, provide an empirical basis for deriving appropriate intervention, and serve as an ongoing evaluation of therapy (Singh et al. 1991). Over the years, assessment methodologies have changed in the field of psychiatry. This is very much reflected in the changing nature of services offered by medical professionals and their diagnostic methods. In the early part of the century, the guiding principle in the care of people with learning disability was symptom management (Weisblatt 1994). This is evident in the medical model of learning disability that prevailed during that time, which largely led to the overuse of medication in people with learning disabilities, and they were viewed as patients regardless of their health status (Mittler 1979).

In so doing, the psychiatric treatment of people with learning disabilities largely consisted of sedation and restraint. Many records show that this treatment was often applied whether or not the person had a co-morbid mental disorder. During the past 20 years, the philosophy of care for people with learning disabilities has emphasised maximising the individual's potential through habilitation approaches and this clearly warrants appropriate and accurate assessment and diagnosis of mental health disorder in this population.

Historically, the central issue in the assessment of dual diagnosis was to distinguish between primary and secondary handicaps (Cutts 1957). Thus professionals examined questions such as does the person have a primary learning disability or is the person primarily mentally ill? And did the mental illness cause learning disability or did the learning disability lead to mental illness? However, the criteria for making the distinction were poorly defined. Reiss (1993) argued that the identification of primary diagnosis can have implications for services: people diagnosed as having learning disability may access learning disability services and those diagnosed as mentally ill are referred to the mental health sector. However, this method is not followed in the diagnostic process and in therapeutic services and traditional diagnostic methods are continued.

Traditionally, American psychiatrists have used the *Diagnostic and Statistical Manual of Mental Disorders* (DSM-IV) for the diagnosis of mental illness in the general population and in people with learning disability (American Psychiatric Association 1994), DSM-IV-TR (American Psychiatric Association 2000) being the most recent version. In Europe, psychiatrists use the International Classification of Diseases, ICD-10 (World Health Organization 1993). These signify the attempts made to apply diagnostic categories from traditional psychiatry. The parallelism and overlap of the ICD-10 and the DSM-IV suggest that consensus may be developing with respect to a universal, international system of psychiatric diagnosis (Febrega 1994).

Diagnostic classifications

DSM-IV defines a mental disorder as 'a clinically significant behavioural or psychological syndrome or pattern associated with personal distress *or* disability (i.e. impairment in one or more important areas of functioning), *or* significant increased risk of suffering pain, disability or important loss of freedom; sexual promiscuity, alcohol or drug dependency, sexual deviance or offending behaviour by itself is NOT a mental disorder, but mental retardation is.'

Enfield and Aman (1995) proposed the following broad definition of what constitutes a psychiatric disorder: 'where behaviour and emotions are abnormal by virtue of their qualitative or quantitative deviance, and cannot be explained on the basis of developmental delay alone, and cause significant distress to the person, carers, or community, as well as significant added impairment.'

The applicability of the psychiatric classification system to people with learning disability has been questioned and various modifications suggested (Campbell and Malone 1991). Indeed both ICD-9 and DSM-III criteria were applied to people with learning disability without alterations or with only minor modification. In people with severe learning disability, the utility of these criteria is doubtful in making a diagnosis of mental health disorder (Ballinger et al. 1991; Dosen 1993).

Sturmey (1995) explored the use of the DSM-III Revised (DSM-III-R) version in people with learning disabilities. This, along with the evidence from a number of studies, demonstrated that people with learning disabilities can display the full range of psychopathology (Rutter and Graham 1970; Eaton and Menolascino 1982; Jacobson 1990) and thus DSM-III-R could be used in this population. However, Sturmey stresses that there are several potential problems in these studies, as many of them are based on psychiatrists' own modified versions of the diagnostic criteria. Both Zimmerman et al. (1986) and Sturmey (1995) argue that these modifications are problematic since they are not always clearly operationalised and lead to substantial changes in the diagnostic process, hence the need for further research in the use of modified criteria in clinical practice.

From a clinical diagnostic perspective, Cooper and Callacott (1994) argue that it is 'naive' to conclude that the lack of standard criteria precludes the diagnosis of an illness. They point out that ICD-10 provides guidelines rather than operational criteria and this encourages 'sensible diagnosis in clinical practice' (p. 401). Although this approach takes a pragmatic view in diagnosing mental disorder, the lack of adherence to standardised criteria in clinical practice leads to reduced reliability and generalisability of the diagnosis.

In response to the criticism of lack of applicability of diagnostic criteria derived from the general population to adults with learning disability, the Royal College of Psychiatrists published DC-LD (*Diagnostic Criteria for Psychiatric Disorders for Use with Adults with Learning Disabilities/Mental Retardation*) (2001). DC-LD it is hoped could be viewed as a 'stand-alone' classificatory system for use with adults with moderate to profound learning disabilities. However, its use is seen as complementary to the ICD-10 manuals for people with mild learning disabilities. In 2003, a supplement of the *Journal of Intellectual Disability Research* (*JIDR*) brought together a series of interesting papers that informed the development of DC-LD, which the interested reader can refer to for further information (September 2003, Vol. 47).

DC-LD structure

DC-LD adopts a hierarchical multi-axial approach to classification. Axes I and II use ICD-10 categories:

- Severity of person's intellectual disabilities (mental retardation) (axis I)
- Cause of a person's intellectual disabilities (axis II)
- Presence of additional psychiatric disorders (axis III)

Axis III is further subdivided into levels A to E as follows:

- Pervasive developmental disorders (axis III level A)
- Psychiatric illness (axis III level B)
- Personality disorder (axis III level C)
- Problem behaviours (axis III level D)
- Other disorders (axis III level E)

The criteria within the above categories are operationalised and incorporate existing clinical and research knowledge concerning the impact of learning disabilities on the nature and presentation of symptoms and signs of mental disorders. If the above approach proves to be clinically useful a further step would be development of rating scales or checklists to generate DC-LD diagnostic categories for clinical and research use.

Diagnostic phenomena

Even at the best of times, the use of diagnostic criteria for mental health disorders in the general population has been questioned. The assessment of mental illness in people with learning disabilities may be confusing, and there is a tendency to underdiagnose or underestimate mental health disorders in this population (Spengler et al. 1990; Sovner and Pary 1993). Hence, during the assessment of dual diagnosis, it is important to avoid diagnostic overshadowing (Reiss et al. 1982). This refers to instances in which the presence of learning disability decreases the diagnostic significance of an accompanying mental health disorder.

Because of learning disability, some debilitating emotional problems may appear less significant than they are when compared to the effects of learning disability. In this context, Reiss (1993) suggests that some form of challenging behaviour or behaviour problems that are viewed as signs of mental health disorders in non-learning disabled people may be viewed as consequences of learning disability. This may not be because of any evidence supporting the attribution, but because of a natural tendency to attribute behaviour to salient factors associated with learning disability.

In a series of studies, Reiss et al. (1982) and Sovner and DesNoyers-Hurley (1986) demonstrated that the same case description of challenging behaviour was rated lower on brief descriptors of psychopathology for a person with learning disability than for a person with an IQ in the average range. However, the saliency hypothesis, which proposed that diagnostic overshadowing would decrease as a function of an increase in IQ, was not well supported by the study of Spengler et al. (1990). They showed that diagnostic overshadowing occurred when IQs of 58 were reported, but not when IQs of 70 or 80 were reported. Based on this observation, they concluded that overshadowing bias appears to be a robust phenomenon for IQs in the low range of moderate learning disability. However, this may not be generalised in people with borderline and mild learning disabilities.

This is further supported by a meta-analysis relating to diagnostic overshadowing by White et al. (1995), in which they concluded that the phenomenon of diagnostic overshadowing does occur in well replicated analogue experiments. This report suggests that various factors such as clinician or situational variables may contribute to the process of diagnostic overshadowing. However, further research is required for any firm conclusion on the influence of these variables.

The hierarchical system of classification as proposed in DC-LD is one way of avoiding diagnostic overshadowing by asking the clinician to complete information about each of the proposed axes separately. Thus using this approach to enable a comprehensive diagnostic formulation, one would need to consider severity of learning disability, additional developmental disorders, such as autistic spectrum disorders, additional psychiatric illness, personality disorder, behavioural phenotypes, problem behaviours and medical conditions. By considering how far each of these categories explains the clinical presentation partially or fully this enables a more holistic approach to clinical assessment and formulation. A standardised system such as this helps to collate information in a structured and systematic way, thus making sharing of information between clinicians and researchers more meaningful and reliable.

Assessment of psychopathology

DesNoyers-Hurley and Silka (2003) note that developmentally appropriate phenomena such as talking to oneself, solitary fantasy play and imaginary friends can easily be mistaken or misinterpreted as symptoms of a psychotic illness in a person with learning disabilities. The overlap of behaviour problems associated with psychopathology poses a further serious challenge to psychiatrists and other professionals involved in diagnosis of mental health disorder in people with learning disabilities. Fraser et al. (1986) stress that the behavioural disturbances seen and commonly identified in people with learning disabilities may be due to any or all of the psychiatric disorders. These include aggressive conduct, mood disturbances, withdrawal, antisocial conduct and self-injurious behaviour (Fraser et al. 1986). Yet, the task of differentiating mental health disorder from any form of challenging behaviour in a person with learning disability is a difficult one. This inability to differentiate between these two aspects is possibly attributed to the modes of presentation, which are common for both. For example, repetitive behaviour by a person with learning disability might be indicative of obsessive–compulsive disorder and hyperactivity might be associated with mania.

When assessing patterns of symptomatology in people with dual diagnosis, Reiss (1993) suggests that it is not essential for every symptom to be present and that a diagnosis can be made if there is a preponderance of relevant symptoms. Reiss further argues that a behaviour problem on its own is insufficient evidence of psychopathology, but it could be one of the symptoms in an overall pattern for arriving at a conclusion of underlying mental health disorder. For example, poor physical hygiene could be part of an entire pattern of psychotic symptoms that is recognised as schizophrenia if a person also shows bizarre behaviour, delusions, hallucinations, avoidance of others and inappropriate emotions.

Reiss further suggests that while assessing psychopathology in people with a learning disability, it is important to make allowances for the individual's learning disability and the circumstances under which he or she lives. Hence, it is vital to examine the physical and social environment of a person with a learning disability in order to aid the process of assessment of challenging behaviour or mental health disorder. Sometimes these people express symptoms in poorly disguised ways, which clouds the assessment process. Therefore, people who are dually diagnosed are frequent victims of errors of both commission and omission (Enfield 1992), which lead to the overprescription of phenothiazines with inadequate indication and the failure to consider diagnoses other than learning disability as the cause of behavioural symptoms. Another issue that affects the diagnosis and prescription of inappropriate medication or the continuation of it is the process of differential diagnosis, which is considered in the section 'Multiple diagnostic presentations and differential diagnosis' (see later in this chapter).

The difficulties of diagnosing mental health disorders in people with learning disability led Sovner and Pary (1993, pp. 94–95) to define the variables that confound the diagnostic process in people with learning disabilities (Box 4.1).

Box 4.1 Diagnostic factors for people with learning disabilities.

(1) *Intellectual distortion*, which is the difficulty the individuals have in communicating their internal feeling state due to concrete thinking, decreased intellect and impaired communication.

(2) *Psychosocial masking*, which describes the impoverished social skills and life experiences that are typical of the population, wherein a psychiatric symptom may not be as 'rich' and detailed as in a person without such disabilities.

(3) *Cognitive disintegration*, which is the lowered threshold, in people with learning disability, for anxiety to become overwhelming and this can present as bizarre behaviour and symptoms that can be mistaken for schizophrenia.

(4) *Baseline exaggeration*, which describes the increase in pre-existing cognitive deficits and maladaptive behaviours which can worsen as a result of the superimposed mental disorder, making the diagnosis more difficult.

These factors along with the evidence from other studies clarify some of the difficulties of diagnosing mental health disorders in people with learning disabilities using psychiatric interviews or checklists alone. Such approaches do not provide the historical context in which the symptoms developed and their progression over time and information about possible causes of the symptoms. The way a mental disorder presents depends on the interaction of a variety of factors, including the articulation and expression of thoughts and feelings and behavioural expression of mental phenomena. Due to the difficulty of obtaining an accurate account of the mental or psychological state from people with learning disabilities, the trend over the last decade has been to rely on third-party reports of the person's behaviour and mental state (Sturmey et al. 1991).

The difficulty of detecting and diagnosing mental health disorders in people with learning disabilities has led to the development of brief questionnaires and rating scales to enhance the diagnostic process (see Appendix 1).

Diagnosis of common mental disorders

The most common types of mental illness found in people with learning disabilities are anxiety disorders, affective disorders such as bipolar disorders and depression, schizophrenia, dementia and personality disorders.

Anxiety disorders

In the general population in the USA, one in four people were found to suffer from anxiety disorder in their lifetime (Kessler et al. 1994). Although anxiety disorders are among the most common psychiatric disorders in the general population, very little is known about the incidence of these disorders in people with a learning disability (Ollendick and Ollendick 1982). According to Fraser and Nolan (1994), acute anxiety states may develop in people with a learning disability as a response to stress, in the same way as in people without any learning disability. However, the expression of these may take different forms in people who have the ability to express their thoughts and feeling either verbally or non-verbally. It is reported that neurotic disorders are characterised by disproportionate levels of anxiety, fearfulness and depression (Day 1985). It is also thought that some degree of worry and stress, which are not disorders as such, are widely experienced by people with learning disabilities (Fraser and Nolan 1994).

Panic disorder

The essential features are recurrent attacks of severe anxiety (panic) which are not restricted to any particular situation or set of circumstances, and which are therefore unpredictable. As in other anxiety disorders, the dominant symptoms vary from person to person, but sudden onset of palpitations, chest pain, choking sensations, dizziness and feelings of unreality (depersonalisation or derealisation) are common. There is also, almost invariably, a secondary fear of dying, losing control or going mad. Individual attacks usually last for minutes only, though sometimes longer; their frequency and the course of the disorder are both rather variable. An individual in a panic attack often experiences a crescendo of fear and autonomic symptoms, which results in an exit, usually hurried, from wherever he or she may be. If this occurs in a specific situation, such as on a bus or in a crowd, the patient may subsequently avoid that situation. Similarly, frequent and unpredictable panic attacks produce fear of being alone or going into public places. A panic attack is often followed by a persistent fear of having another attack. For a definite diagnosis, several severe attacks of autonomic anxiety should have occurred within a period of about one month.

Agoraphobia

Most sufferers of agoraphobia are women and the onset is usually early in adult life. Depressive and obsessional symptoms and social phobias may also be present but do not dominate the clinical picture. In the absence of effective treatment, agoraphobia often becomes chronic, usually with a fluctuating course over time.

All of the following criteria should be fulfilled in order to make a definite diagnosis of agoraphobia:

- The psychological or autonomic symptoms must be primarily manifestations of anxiety and not secondary to other symptoms, such as delusions or obsessional thoughts.
- The anxiety must be restricted to (or occur mainly in) at least two of the following situations: crowds, public places, travelling away from home and travelling alone.
- Avoidance of the phobic situation must be, or must have been, a prominent feature.

Social phobia

Social phobias often start in adolescence and are centred on a fear of scrutiny by other people in comparatively small groups (as opposed to crowds), leading to avoidance of social situations. Unlike most other phobias, social phobias are equally common in men and women. They may be discrete (for example restricted to eating in public, to public speaking or to encounters with the opposite sex) or diffuse, involving almost all social situations outside the family circle. A fear of vomiting in public may be important. Social phobias are usually associated with low self-esteem and fear of criticism. They may present as a complaint of blushing, hand tremor, nausea or urgency of micturition, the individual sometimes being convinced that one of these secondary manifestations of anxiety is the primary problem; symptoms may progress to panic attacks. Avoidance is often marked, and in extreme cases may result in almost complete social isolation.

Specific (isolated) phobias

These are phobias restricted to highly specific situations, such as proximity to particular animals, heights, thunder, darkness, flying, closed spaces, urinating or defecating in public toilets, eating certain foods, dentistry, the sight of blood or injury or the fear of exposure to specific diseases. Although the triggering situation is discrete, contact with it can evoke panic, as in agoraphobia and social phobias. Specific phobias usually arise in childhood or early adult life and can persist for decades if they remain untreated. The seriousness of the resulting handicap depends on how easy it is for the sufferer to avoid the phobic situation. Fear of the phobic situation tends not to fluctuate, in contrast to agoraphobia. Radiation sickness and venereal infections and, more recently, AIDS are common subjects of disease phobias.

Generalised anxiety disorder

The essential feature is anxiety, which is generalised and persistent but not restricted to, or even strongly predominating in, any particular environmental circumstances (i.e. it is 'free-floating'). As in other anxiety disorders, the dominant symptoms are highly variable, but complaints of continuous feelings of nervousness, trembling, muscular tension, sweating, lightheadedness, palpitations, dizziness and epigastric discomfort are common. Fears that the sufferer or a relative will shortly become ill or have an accident are often expressed, together with a variety of other worries and foreboding. This disorder is more common in women, and often related to chronic environmental stress. Its course is variable but tends to be fluctuating and chronic.

Obsessive–compulsive disorder (OCD)

The essential feature of this disorder is recurrent obsessional thoughts or compulsive acts. (For brevity, 'obsessional' will be used subsequently in place of 'obsessive–compulsive' when referring to symptoms.) Obsessional thoughts are ideas, images or impulses that enter the individual's mind again and again in a stereotyped form. They are almost invariably distressing (because they are violent or obscene, or simply because they are perceived as senseless) and the sufferer often tries, unsuccessfully, to resist them. They are, however, recognised as the individual's own thoughts, even though they are involuntary and often repugnant. Compulsive acts or rituals are stereotyped behaviours that are repeated again and again. They are not inherently enjoyable, nor do they result in the completion of inherently useful tasks. The individual often views them as preventing some objectively unlikely event, often involving harm to or caused by himself or herself. Usually, though not invariably, the individual recognises this behaviour as pointless or ineffectual and repeated attempts are made to resist it; in very long-standing cases, resistance may be minimal. Autonomic anxiety symptoms are often present, and distressing feelings of internal or psychic tension without obvious autonomic arousal are also common. There is a close relationship between obsessional symptoms, particularly obsessional thoughts, and depression. Individuals with OCD often have depressive symptoms, and patients suffering from recurrent depressive disorder may develop obsessional thoughts during episodes of depression. In either situation, an increase or decrease in the severity of the depressive symptoms is generally accompanied by a parallel change in the severity of the obsessional symptoms.

OCD is equally common in men and women, and there are often prominent anankastic features in the underlying personality. Onset is usually in childhood or early adult life. The course is variable and more likely to be chronic in the absence of significant depressive symptoms. The stories of Nigel and Debi illustrate the impact of obsessional behaviours in people with learning disabilities.

Nigel is a 21-year-old with mild learning disabilities, who currently works at a supermarket. Nigel's problems involve compulsive hand washing and fear of contamination with germs. Thus Nigel has to wear gloves when he is at work. He has rituals about what he will touch and what he will avoid. When washing his hands he will first dig his nails into the soap bar and then wash his hands without touching the sink or taps. He would not use a cloth towel to dry his hands, instead he uses paper towels. His obsessional symptoms are affecting his work. In the past he also used to have rituals about washing his face in a certain way. This appears to have improved over time. Clinically the diagnosis appears to be an OCD. Further assessment by a community nurse from the learning disability team as well as a clinical psychologist would be helpful to identify the triggers of Nigel's behaviour and to devise an appropriate behavioural plan to reduce his compulsive behaviour.

Debi is 23 years of age with Down's syndrome, ritualistic behaviour and obsessions concerning personal cleanliness following use of the toilet. Debi lives at home and attends the day centre 5 days a week. However, she is missing the majority of the sessions as she can be in the toilet for up to 2 to 3 hours. This behaviour also results in her missing or delaying the transport home. Recently, Debi blocked two toilets at the day centre, causing flooding. Her placement at the centre is at risk. Her OCD was assessed using the compulsive behaviour checklist. Debi arranges clothes in a parallel way, arranges toilet rolls and insists on a rigid daily routine. She also insists on doing her own shoelaces and personal hygiene, even though she takes a long time over it. She cleans her body parts excessively, especially hands and face, which is causing skin problems. Debi's compulsive behaviour is interfering with her daily routine and with her social activities and relationships with others.

Diagnostic guidelines of OCD

For a definite diagnosis, obsessional symptoms or compulsive acts, or both, must be present on most days for at least two successive weeks and be a source of distress or interference with activities. The obsessional symptoms should have the following characteristics:

- They must be recognised as the individual's own thoughts or impulses.
- There must be at least one thought or act that is still resisted unsuccessfully, even though others may be present that the sufferer no longer resists.
- The thought of carrying out the act must not in itself be pleasurable (simple relief of tension or anxiety is not regarded as pleasure in this sense).
- The thoughts, images or impulses must be unpleasantly repetitive.

(To elicit the above good verbal communication is required.)

Post-traumatic stress disorder (PTSD)

This arises as a delayed and/or protracted response to a stressful event or situation (either short- or long-lasting) of an exceptionally threatening or catastrophic nature, which is likely to cause pervasive distress in almost anyone (for example natural or man-made disaster, combat, serious accident, witnessing the violent death of others, or being the victim of torture, terrorism, rape or other crime). Predisposing factors such as personality traits (e.g. compulsive, asthenic) or previous history of neurotic illness may lower the threshold for the development of the syndrome or aggravate its course, but they are neither necessary nor sufficient to explain its occurrence.

Typical symptoms include episodes of repeated reliving of the trauma in intrusive memories ('flashbacks') or dreams, occurring against the persisting background of a sense of 'numbness' and emotional blunting, detachment from other people, unresponsiveness to surroundings, anhedonia and avoidance of activities and situations reminiscent of the trauma. Commonly there is fear and avoidance of cues that remind the sufferer of the original trauma. Rarely, there may be dramatic, acute bursts of fear, panic or aggression, triggered by stimuli arousing a sudden recollection and/or re-enactment of the trauma or of the original reaction to it.

There is usually a state of autonomic hyperarousal with hypervigilance, an enhanced startle reaction and insomnia. Anxiety and depression are commonly associated with the above symptoms and signs, and suicidal ideation is not infrequent. Excessive use of alcohol or drugs may be a complicating factor.

The onset follows the trauma with a latency period, which may range from a few weeks to months (but rarely exceeds 6 months). The course is fluctuating, but recovery can be expected in the majority of cases. In a small proportion of patients the condition may show a chronic course over many years and a transition to an enduring personality change.

According to ICD-10 diagnostic guidelines, this disorder should not generally be diagnosed unless there is evidence that it arose within six months of a traumatic event of exceptional severity. A 'probable' diagnosis might still be possible if the delay between the event and the onset was longer than 6 months, provided that the clinical manifestations are typical and no alternative identification of the disorder (for example as an anxiety disorder, OCD or depressive episode) is plausible. In addition to evidence of trauma, there must be a repetitive, intrusive recollection or re-enactment of the event in memories, daytime imagery or dreams. Conspicuous emotional detachment, numbing of feeling and avoidance of stimuli that might arouse recollection of the trauma are often present but are not essential for the diagnosis. The autonomic disturbances, mood disorder and behavioural abnormalities all contribute to the diagnosis but are not of prime importance.

PTSD in adults with learning disabilities

There is limited literature on the subject of PTSD in people with learning disability. The following story highlights the nature of PTSD in a person with moderate learning disabilities.

Sudha is a 19-year-old South Asian woman with Down's syndrome and moderate learning disabilities. She lives with her mother and brother; her parents were divorced about 14 years ago. Sudha's mother works part-time. Sudha alleged that at the age of 16 she was sexually abused in a respite home, by a carer. Since then her mother has observed behavioural changes, which have worsened with time. Sudha has been observed talking to walls and nodding and laughing as if someone was talking to her. She talks to herself even when watching TV. Her mother reports that this was not observed prior to the alleged abuse. Her mother had overheard her saying, 'Get off', and moving her body away as if someone was hurting her. This appears to occur usually when Sudha is in bed at night. Her mother has also heard her saying, 'Get out' when in her room. Sudha has been observed standing in front of a mirror and talking to her image. When travelling in the car she has been behaving as if the dashboard was talking to her. She had also been insisting that the bathroom door and her mother's bedroom door be kept open. She did not give any reason for this apart from saying it is 'private'. On one occasion she got up in the middle of the night and tried to run away. She gives no reason for her odd behaviour, but repeatedly commented 'it is private' when questioned.

According to her mother, the most distressing problem was her behaviour of talking to herself. She appeared to be talking to 'imaginary friends' who seemed to be abusive towards her. She did not have such imaginary friends before the alleged assault. Sudha had at times been found in a panic state, claiming that there was smoke or fire in her room. She had also become obsessed with a teacher, Miss Nair. She once stole the teacher's photograph, glasses, a CD and other personal papers and brought them home. She had been observed speaking to the teacher's photograph. She had also written notes to Miss Nair. Sudha had developed sleeping difficulty since the onset of the above symptoms. Her appetite had not changed. Her mother observed that in the past few years she has become more withdrawn and has lost interest in pleasurable activities such as going to the gym and swimming. She used to enjoy such activities before the alleged assault. She had lost friends, becoming 'moody' and 'irritable' and was no longer interested in going out. Sudha had been found with a dressing cord around her neck on three occasions. Fortunately the cord was not tied tightly. She was once found choking on a bottle. It was unclear whether this was a self-harm attempt or an accident. At times, Sudha had started pretending that she had hurt herself and would put tissue around her wrists. Occasionally she fell to the floor deliberately shouting 'Stop it, get off' as if someone had thrown her down and was hurting her.

An assessment by a child psychiatrist confirmed that Sudha had symptoms suggestive of PTSD and that it was unlikely she was suffering from a psychotic illness. It was also noted that on occasions Sudha had been 'sexually disinhibited', pulling her pants down and pelvic thrusting against objects.

McCarthy (2001) in her review of PTSD in learning disabilities emphasises that the clinician needs to be aware that PTSD should be considered in the differential diagnosis of a person with learning disability presenting with a wide array of symptoms, for example aggression, disruptive or defiant behaviour, self-harm, agitation or jumpiness, distractibility, sleeping problems and depressed mood. McCarthy states that there has been only one reported major study of adults with learning disability who were diagnosed with PTSD (Ryan 1994). 'This was of a clinic population of 51 adults and showed that people with learning disability develop PTSD at a rate comparable to the able population when exposed to trauma. Each person had suffered at least two types of trauma. That most frequently experienced was sexual abuse by multiple perpetrators (commonly starting in childhood), physical abuse or life-threatening neglect committed with some other active abuse or trauma. A few cases did not involve abuse: for example, a sibling dying in a fire, seeing a close friend die during a seizure or an accident or witnessing a parent commit suicide by a gunshot wound to the head. All those cases of trauma involved seeing a carer, friend or close relative die in traumatic circumstances. Almost all those with PTSD were referred with violent or disruptive behaviour. The most common psychiatric diagnosis prior to the diagnosis of PTSD was no diagnosis or schizophrenia. Other more common diagnoses included autism and intermittent explosive disorder. In about half of the cases someone working with the client knew of the traumatic event. The most common co morbid psychiatric condition diagnosed when PTSD was identified was a major depression.'

Diagnostic issues of anxiety disorders in learning disabilities

Bailey and Andrews (2003) suggest that there is little doubt that adults with learning difficulties can suffer from a wide range of anxiety disorders. There is considerable variation in the reported rates of such disorders, ranging from 0.6 to 57%. Many studies do not make a definite diagnosis but report anxiety symptoms, the prevalence of which varied from 6 to 31%. With more severe learning disabilities only behavioural symptoms can be assessed reliably, thus making it more difficult for all the criteria of an anxiety disorder to be met. There is widespread acknowledgement about the difficulties of using diagnostic criteria developed for the general population in adults with learning disabilities. Anxiety is a normal phenomenon and an adaptive response to daily stressors and threats. Thus it can be difficult to decide when anxiety becomes pathological for a given person in his or her particular circumstances. This is made even more difficult in a person who has limited ability to describe complex internal experiences and thus more reliance has to be given to reports from others who know the person well. When fears are expressed by a person with learning disabilities one also needs to consider whether such fears are developmentally appropriate. Research suggests that fears of adults with learning difficulties are similar to those reported by children of equivalent developmental age, for example fears of ghosts, thunder and animals. Whether such a fear is considered pathological would depend on both the content, severity and persistence as well as the intensity of distress caused to the person and its impact on his/her social functioning.

The evaluation, diagnosis and treatment of any form of mental health disorder in people with a learning disability require the expertise and teamwork of all professionals involved. In clinical practice, often there is a tendency by carers to ignore or underestimate the importance of anxiety symptoms expressed by people with a learning disability (Patel et al. 1993). It is believed that anxiety disorders and OCD are diagnosed less frequently in people with a learning disability (Vitello and Behar 1992). There is a tendency to assume that inappropriate or strange behavioural patterns are a manifestation of developmental delay rather than an indication of an accompanying mental health disorder.

OCD is often confused with stereotypic behaviours. Of course, this may be true of other types of anxiety disorders as well. Early detection of stress reactions by carers can often prevent these leading to full-blown anxiety disorders. This could be conducted through comprehensive assessment of a person's behaviour and mental state using a range of measures, such as standardised psychiatric interview, use of custom-made checklists for anxiety symptoms, nursing care plans and accurate recording and teamwork by a range of service agencies (Raghavan 1998). In addition to these, the use of rating scales such as the Zung Self-Rating Anxiety Scale (Zung 1965), the Reiss Screen for Maladaptive Behaviour (Reiss 1988) and the Compulsive Behaviour Checklist developed by Gedye (Gedye 1992) could assist clinicians in assessing compulsive behaviours in people with learning disabilities.

Affective disorders

Affective disorders are a group of mental disturbances characterised by specific abnormalities of mood in association with alterations in cognition, behaviour and physical functioning (Synder 1988; Sovner and Pary 1993). They are referred to as mood disorders, of which the two main types are depression and mania. Until recently, it was relatively common to question the possibility that people with a learning disability could develop an affective disorder (Sovner and Pary 1993). However, now it has become apparent that, like other mental disorders, people with a learning disability can manifest the full range of affective disorders, with depressed mood being the most common symptom. According to Reiss and Benson (1985), depression is among the most important topics in the study of mental health aspects of learning disability and this is reflected in the large number of papers published in this field.

The major affective disorders include bipolar disorder and major depression, which are distinguished on the basis of whether or not a manic episode has ever occurred. It is suggested that depression is more common than mania (Tomb 1992). In his studies Reid (1985) found that in people with learning disabilities affective disorder may present either as a single episode or as a relapsing condition with recurrent episodes of depression or mania or both.

According to ICD-10 diagnostic guidelines, in these disorders the fundamental disturbance is a change in affect or mood to either low mood (depression) or elation. Some people may experience a single depressive episode in their lifetime. Others commonly experience recurrent depressive episodes, the so-called recurrent depressive disorder. The term bipolar affective disorder is applied to those who have had episodes of elation (hypomania/mania) in addition to episodes of depression. Sometimes individuals may experience mixed affective states in which symptoms of depression are simultaneously present with symptoms of mania, with neither symptom type predominating. Mixed affective episodes appear to occur more commonly among adults with learning disabilities than they do among the general population (Royal College of Psychiatrists 2001).

Hypomania

Hypomania is a lesser degree of mania. There is a persistent mild elevation of mood (for at least several days on end), increased energy and activity, and usually marked feelings of well-being and both physical and mental efficiency.

Increased sociability, talkativeness, overfamiliarity, increased sexual libido and a decreased need for sleep are often present, but not to the extent that they lead to severe disruption of work or result in social rejection. Irritability, conceit and boorish behaviour may take the place of the more usual euphoric sociability.

Concentration and attention may be impaired, thus diminishing the ability to settle down to work or to relaxation and leisure, but this may not prevent the appearance of interests in new ventures and activities, or overspending.

Mania

This is a more severe disorder where the mood is elevated out of keeping with the individual's circumstances and may vary from carefree joviality to almost uncontrollable excitement. Elation is accompanied by increased energy, resulting in overactivity, pressure of speech and a decreased need for sleep. Normal social inhibitions are lost, attention cannot be sustained and there is often marked distractibility. Self-esteem is inflated, and grandiose or overoptimistic ideas are freely expressed.

Perceptual disorders may occur, such as the appreciation of colours as especially vivid (and usually beautiful), a preoccupation with the fine details of surfaces or textures, and subjective hyperacusis (painful sensitivity to sounds). The individual may embark on extravagant and impractical schemes, spend money recklessly or become aggressive, amorous or facetious in inappropriate circumstances. In some manic episodes the mood is irritable and suspicious rather than elated. The peak age of onset for mania is 15 to 30 years, but the first episode may occur at any age from late childhood to the seventh or eighth decade.

Diagnostic guidelines for mania

The episode should last for at least one week and should be severe enough to disrupt ordinary work and social activities more or less completely. The mood change should be accompanied by increased energy and several of the symptoms referred to above (particularly pressure of speech, decreased need for sleep, grandiosity and excessive optimism).

Bipolar affective disorder

This disorder is characterised by repeated (at least two) episodes in which the patient's mood and activity levels are significantly disturbed, this disturbance consisting on some occasions of an elevation of mood and increased energy and activity (mania or hypomania), and on others of a lowering of mood and decreased energy and activity (depression). Characteristically, recovery is usually complete between episodes, and the incidence in the two sexes is more nearly equal than in other mood disorders.

Depression

The individual usually suffers from depressed mood, loss of interest and enjoyment, and reduced energy leading to increased fatigue and diminished activity. Marked tiredness after only slight effort is common. Other symptoms include:

- Reduced concentration and attention
- Reduced self-esteem and self-confidence
- Ideas of guilt and unworthiness (even in a mild type of episode)
- Bleak and pessimistic views of the future
- Ideas or acts of self-harm or suicide
- Disturbed sleep
- Diminished appetite

The lowered mood varies little from day to day, and is often unresponsive to circumstances, yet may show a characteristic diurnal variation, improving as the day goes on. As with manic episodes, the clinical presentation shows marked individual variations, and atypical presentations are particularly common in adolescents and in adults with learning disabilities. In some cases, anxiety, distress and motor agitation may be more prominent. Other prominent symptoms may be irritability, excessive consumption of alcohol, histrionic behaviour, mood swings or hypochondriacal preoccupations. Exacerbation of pre-existing phobic or obsessional symptoms may also mask the depression. For depressive episodes, a duration of at least 2 weeks is usually required for diagnosis, but shorter periods may be reasonably acknowledged if symptoms are unusually severe and of rapid onset.

Some of the above symptoms may be marked and develop characteristic features that are widely regarded as having special clinical significance. The most typical examples of these are 'somatic' symptoms: loss of interest or pleasure in activities that are normally enjoyable; lack of emotional reactivity to normally pleasurable surroundings and events; waking in the morning 2 hours or more before the usual time; depression worse in the morning; objective evidence of psychomotor retardation or agitation (remarked on or reported by other people); marked loss of appetite; weight loss (often defined as 5% or more of body weight in the past month); and marked loss of libido.

In very severe depression, delusions, hallucinations or depressive stupor may sometimes be present. The delusions usually involve ideas of sin, poverty or imminent disaster, responsibility for which may be assumed by the patient. Auditory or olfactory (smell) hallucinations are usually of defamatory or accusatory voices or of rotting filth or decomposing flesh. Severe psychomotor retardation may progress to stupor.

Diagnostic issues of affective disorders in learning disabilities

Standard general population diagnostic criteria such as ICD-10 and DSM-IV-TR are difficult to apply fully to people with severe and profound learning disabilities. For example, a full understanding of complex concepts such as guilt and worthlessness requires a developmental level of about 7 years. Those without verbal communication skills would be unable to report recurrent thoughts of death or suicidal ideation or diminished ability to think, therefore limiting the usefulness of such criteria (Smiley and Cooper 2003).

McCraken and Diamond (1988) in their report of five cases of bipolar illness in adolescents with a learning disability suggest that bipolar illness is commonly misdiagnosed in this population because of difficulties in eliciting histories of mood change and overemphasis on psychotic and pseudo-organic symptoms. In people with learning disability, depressive disorder may be difficult to diagnose because of impaired communication and the modifying effects of underlying brain damage (Yappa and Roy 1990). There is also reason to believe that depression is significantly underdiagnosed, as the person with learning disability has reduced ability to disclose his or her own mood, and the psychiatrist is thereby denied access to the cardinal symptoms of affective illness (Enfield 1992).

Often people with mild learning disability may be able to report their thoughts, feelings and emotions to another person, but in the case of people with severe learning disability, the psychiatrist must often rely on non-verbal cues from the client and behavioural observations from carers. In many cases, symptoms such as reduced psychomotor activity, weight loss and sad facial expressions may be seen as non-disruptive, which lessens the likelihood that these clinical signs are regarded as problems by carers. The fact that many individuals receive psychiatric diagnoses based on informants' reports of symptoms may account for at least some degree of the present underreporting of depression in this population (Enfield 1992).

Enfield (1992) further argues that mania tends to be overdiagnosed, as overactivity and excitement are common symptoms in this population. Charlot et al. (1993) suggest that as clinicians become more sensitive to the concern of overdiagnosis of mania, a downward trend in its occurrence might be expected. Another major issue is the lack of diagnostic criteria for depression in people with learning disability. However, it has been reported that the pragmatic application of standardised diagnostic criteria could to an extent overcome this problem.

Indeed, studies by Meins (1995) and Marston et al. (1997) suggest that standardised diagnostic criteria, such as DSM-IV and ICD-10, can be effectively used to detect depression associated with mild learning disability, but these criteria may be less useful for people with severe learning disability. In the latter group, atypical symptoms may occur, for example irritable or labile mood rather than low mood, or onset or worsening of behavioural problems such as self-injury, screaming and aggression. Reduction in speech output or communication, social withdrawal, increased insecurity with reassurance-seeking behaviour, distress when alone, regression with onset of bed wetting, soiling and increasing dependency on others could also signify a mood disorder.

In some, increased worry about physical health or somatic complaints and worries about serious physical illness may dominate the clinical picture.

Individuals with mood disorder and somatic symptoms are difficult to reassure despite medical investigations that rule out the presence of a serious physical illness. Symptoms that have understandably been found to be uncommon in people with severe learning disabilities include inappropriate guilt, increased self-reproach, recurrent thoughts of death or suicide, complaints of diminished ability to think or concentrate, self-reported indecisiveness, delusions of sin, worthlessness, bodily disease, impending disaster and derisive or condemnatory auditory hallucinations that are in keeping with the low mood. On the other hand the more observable biological symptoms that may be evident in the more severely disabled include changes in energy, sleep disturbance, appetite and/or weight change and excessive restlessness or slowing down, sometimes to the point of complete immobility or stupor.

In order to assist the diagnosis of depression, several rating scales have been used for screening purposes. These include the Beck Depression Inventory (Beck et al. 1961) and Hamilton Depression Rating Scale (Hamilton 1960). Even though clinicians and researchers in this field use many of these scales, studies using a range of these tools to diagnose depression produced disappointing and mixed results in correlating the scores with each other and psychiatric diagnosis (Kazdin et al. 1983; Helsel and Matson 1988).

DC-LD category III-B4.1 depressive episode requires symptoms to be present nearly every day for at least 2 weeks, and at least depressed or irritable mood and/or loss of interest or pleasure in activities, social withdrawal, reduction in self-care or reduction in the quantity of speech or communication to be present. Other additional symptoms that are not included in ICD-10 are an increase in reassurance-seeking behaviour, onset or increase in anxiety or fearfulness, increase in specific problem behaviour and reduced ability to concentrate or distractibility. The ICD-10 items of recurrent suicidal thoughts and inappropriate guilt and worthlessness are not included in DC-LD.

Schizophrenia

Schizophrenia is one of the most distressing of all mental conditions. Not only does it strike young and otherwise fit people, but also it often does so without warning. ICD-10 notes that the schizophrenic disorders are characterised by fundamental and characteristic distortions of thinking and perception and by inappropriate or blunted affect or mood. The main features of this disorder include disturbance of thinking, disturbance of emotions, lack of drive, inactivity, disturbance of motor activity, primary delusions and hallucinations.

There has been renewed interest in the possibility that the relationship between psychosis and intelligence may hold important clues to the aetiology of these disorders (Offord and Cross 1971). It is now well established that schizophrenia is associated with cognitive deficits which may develop many years before the onset of psychosis, and may worsen as the psychosis proceeds. These deficits include impairments of general IQ, attention and working memory. The cognitive deficits overlap with negative symptoms which include marked apathy, paucity of speech, underactivity, blunting of affect, passivity and lack of initiative, and poor non-verbal communication (by facial expression, eye contact, voice modulation and posture). Cognitive deficits and negative symptoms are the most important determinants of the long-term outcome of the illness as regards social functioning. The cognitive impairments also contribute to lack of insight and interfere with psychotherapies that rely upon verbal learning. Epidemiological studies have shown that schizophrenia is three times more likely to occur in those with learning disabilities than in the general population. The reasons for this increase are unclear, leading to several possibilities (Doody et al. 1998). First, schizophrenia in those with learning disabilities may represent a more severe form of the illness. Second, cognitive impairment and the associated deficits of learning disability may make the individual more susceptible to developing the illness. Third, it is possible that a common cause gives rise to both conditions. Repeated replication of the finding that schizophrenia and learning disability occur together more often than chance makes it unlikely that the co-occurrence of both conditions is coincidental (Turner 1989).

Historically, Emil Kraeplin first identified schizophrenia as a distinct disorder. His original term for schizophrenia, dementia praecox, was based on his observations that these patients developed their illness at a relatively early age (praecox) and were likely to have a chronic and deteriorating course (dementia). Kraeplin (1919) first coined the term 'pfropfschizophrenie' to describe dementia praecox occurring with pre-existing intellectual disability. The existence of schizophrenia in people with learning disability has been debated for many years. Beier (1919) suggested that although any type of psychosis may be seen in people with learning disabilities, schizophrenia has the highest incidence of 'common cerebral inferiority'. Beier also held the view that schizophrenia is most commonly associated with learning disability.

The number of papers published with the title of schizophrenia and learning disability is limited in comparison to affective disorder or general issues in dual diagnosis. The published literature points to a difference in the symptoms of schizophrenia between people with learning disability and people of average intelligence (Corbett 1979; Reid 1989; Turner 1989). Reid (1972) emphasised the difficulty of diagnosing catatonic schizophrenia based on stereotypic movement and manneristic behaviour, without access to the patient's mental content. Detailed studies of catatonic symptoms in people with learning disability are lacking in the literature. The following three case histories highlight how schizophrenia manifests in people with learning disabilities.

> Simon is a 65-year-old with moderate learning disabilities, who has been resettled into a group home from a long-stay institution. He has a tendency to talk to himself, has poor motivation, is nervous and does not like crowds

or noise. At the age of 38, he was described as an odd, detached, obsessional, introverted, solitary individual. He needs a good deal of prompting to finish meals, get in and out of bed and dress himself. At times, Simon is overactive, wandering about, very restless and sometimes aggressive towards other residents. He talks in a disjointed manner with inappropriate affect. Simon needs direct supervision whilst washing and bathing. He does not, of his own volition, ask for a change of clothing. He constantly mutters to himself, resists any kind of attention, and becomes verbally hostile towards anyone who he feels is trying to take an interest in him. He giggles for no apparent reason, talking out loud to no one in particular, often talking in vague sentences or in Shakespearean fashion. He says things like, 'Keep quiet' and 'Hurry up'. Sometimes Simon talks of appropriate things, for instance once he complained of lack of privacy. On another occasion, when found to be reading a book and coming down late for breakfast, he said that he was reading as it helped him keep his sanity in this place. Simon likes routine. He takes little interest in any leisure activities. He uses the radio only at specific times throughout the day and will not use it when he has more free time, for example at weekends. He enjoys comedies, especially cartoons on the television. He is reluctant to go on outings with small groups and refuses to go on holidays. Psychiatric diagnosis: chronic schizophrenia with social aloofness, poor motivation, emotional flattening, thought disorder and periodic outbursts in response to hallucinations.

Peter is a 27-year-old with moderate learning disabilities. Peter had a happy childhood and he attended a special school. He was admitted to a ward in a mainstream mental health service from a group home due to his strange behaviour. Psychiatric assessment highlighted his elaborate bizarre delusions and hallucinations, for example he claims he can do black magic, is part of the masters of the universe police force, and can travel between the real world and the spirit world. Mugwai, a martial arts expert from the Peking dynasty, lives inside him and speaks with his voice. Peter is able to demonstrate this by speaking in a guttural tone and saying words that are made up (neologisms) and that do not make any sense. He talks about Morgana, his girlfriend who lives in the spirit world who he met when he 'took out' M, i.e. the master of the universe who had 'put the universe inside him'. He talks about black magic and voodoo influencing him. He experiences passivity phenomena, making him have erections (he says 'It feels like being abused' and so on). Peter's thinking is incoherent and requires repeated clarification to understand what he is trying to say.

Jasmine is a 42-year-old woman with mild learning disabilities. Her first contact with psychiatric services was at the age of 22 due to mental breakdown. She was treated with electroconvulsive therapy (ECT) but had a relapse at the age of 26. Recent admission to a mainstream psychiatric hospital and psychiatric assessment indicated thought disorder, catatonic withdrawal and inability to attend to personal hygiene. Jasmine's skills and abilities gradually declined over a 12 month period according to her mother. Her behaviour became very bizarre and she had odd beliefs; for example, she believed she was working for the police force and also had a job in hospital, and that her mum was stealing her money and rings. She stopped going out of the house and lost a lot of weight due to self-neglect. Jasmine has no insight. She has unrealistic ideas about her ability to care for herself without help and needs prompting with all aspects of care on the ward. She has poor eye contact and a flat, labile mood with tearfulness for no apparent reason. She is perplexed and appears preoccupied with her thoughts. Her speech is vague with jumbled thoughts. She says she does not hear imaginery voices, but appears preoccupied at times as if responding. Jasmine is disoriented regarding time and place, believing she is at home not in hospital.

Diagnostic guidelines for schizophrenia

The schizophrenic disorders are characterised in general by fundamental and characteristic distortions of thinking and perception, and by inappropriate or blunted affect, i.e. mood. Clear consciousness and intellectual capacity are usually maintained, although certain cognitive deficits may evolve in the course of time. The disturbance involves the most basic functions that give the normal person a feeling of individuality, uniqueness and self-direction. The most intimate thoughts, feelings and acts are often felt to be known to or shared by others, and explanatory delusions may develop, to the extent that natural or supernatural forces are believed to be at work influencing the afflicted individual's thoughts and actions in ways that are often bizarre. The individual may see himself or herself as the pivot of all that happens. Hallucinations, especially auditory, are common and may comment on the individual's behaviour or thoughts.

Perception is frequently disturbed in other ways: colours or sounds may seem unduly vivid or altered in quality, and irrelevant features of ordinary things may appear more important than the whole object or situation. Perplexity is also common early on and frequently leads to a belief that everyday situations possess a special, usually sinister, meaning intended uniquely for the individual. In the characteristic schizophrenic disturbance of thinking, peripheral and irrelevant features of a total concept, which are inhibited in normal mental activity, are brought to the fore and utilised in place of those that are relevant and appropriate to the situation. Thus thinking becomes vague, elliptical and obscure, and its expression in speech sometimes incomprehensible. Breaks and interpolations in the train of thought are frequent. There may be complaints that thoughts are being interfered with by an outside agency or power.

Mood is characteristically shallow, flat or incongruous. Ambivalence and disturbance of volition may appear as inertia, negativism or stupor. Catatonia may be present. The onset may be acute, with seriously disturbed behaviour, or insidious, with a gradual development of odd ideas and conduct. The course of the disorder shows equally great variation and is by no means inevitably chronic or deteriorating. In a proportion of cases (15–20%), which may vary in different cultures and populations, the outcome is complete, or nearly complete, recovery. The sexes are approximately equally affected, but the onset tends to be later in women. Men tend to have a poorer long-term outcome than women due to earlier age of onset.

Diagnostic issues of schizophrenia in learning disabilities

The diagnosis of schizophrenia in people with learning disability becomes more difficult as the severity of learning disability increases. These disorders may first present as a change in behaviour, for example the person may become more verbally or physically aggressive, suspicious or socially withdrawn and aloof. He or she may start behaving in an odd or uncharacteristic manner, for example they may become more argumentative or speak to imaginary friends or persecutors. The person's conversation and thought content may become increasingly bizarre and difficult to make sense of. Delusional beliefs may become apparent on further exploration. These are firm unshakeable beliefs, but in a person with learning disability who is suggestible, they may not be held with firm conviction. Thus it may be possible temporarily to talk the person out of his/her beliefs, but he/she may then repeatedly return to the same false belief. An open questioning style is preferable when trying to diagnose schizophrenia as this is less likely to inadvertently suggest symptoms the person may readily agree with, even if such abnormal beliefs or perceptions are absent.

In persons with learning disability it is particularly difficult to elicit passivity phenomena, that is, the belief that an outside agency or alien force is controlling one's thoughts or actions. Similarly even in those with mild learning disability it is particularly difficult to elicit disorders of thought possession, that is, beliefs that alien thoughts are being inserted into one's mind, or that one's thoughts are being withdrawn from the mind or are being broadcast so those nearby who can 'tune into' them and read one's mind. In order to be able to report such phenomena one must be aware of the normal nature of one's thoughts, i.e. that they are personal, confined to the mind and no one else may share them unless the person tells another what he or she is thinking; thus it is impossible for others to 'read' one's mind. Similar considerations apply to hallucinations, that is, perceptions for which there is no objective basis in reality, for example hearing voices when no one is about. Here again the person with learning disability needs to be aware of what is considered abnormal for him/her to realise that hallucinations are abnormal phenomena. The content of hallucinations and delusions may be simple and lack detail or imagination. DC-LD notes that some 'positive' symptoms that are seen in the general population with schizophrenia are uncommonly reported in people with learning disabilities. Examples include delusional perception, passivity phenomena, thought echo, hallucinatory voices giving a running commentary and thought alienation.

It is difficult for us to understand how people with severe or profound learning disability make sense of the world around them. As professionals we cannot assume that our view of what is accepted as normal is also applicable to a person with very limited thinking and cognitive abilities. Thus the diagnosis of schizophrenia in people with learning disability is problematic, as obtaining clear descriptions of first-rank symptoms described above is very difficult except in people with mild or borderline learning disability (Moss et al. 1996). In most people with severe and profound learning disability it is unlikely that schizophrenia could be diagnosed using current criteria. The behaviour of such people is often too primitive and disorganised to allow a diagnosis of schizophrenia. Despite this, there is evidence that schizophrenia is over-diagnosed in this population (Aman et al. 1985) and this may derive from the misdiagnosis of hallucinations (Enfield 1992). Hallucinations are often perceived as voices, familiar and unfamiliar but distinct from the person's own thoughts. James et al. (1996) argues that it may be difficult to know whether people with learning disability are describing vivid thoughts or true hallucinations. Similarly, it may also be difficult to distinguish delusions from strongly held and unusual beliefs. James et al. suggest that as people with learning disability are often closely supervised and spoken about behind their backs, it is important to differentiate delusions from the concerns of people who believe that others are talking about them, laughing at them or secretly observing them.

Negative symptoms of schizophrenia in the general population, which include marked apathy, paucity of speech, underactivity, blunting of affect, passivity and lack of initiative, and poor non-verbal communication (by facial expression, eye contact, voice modulation and posture), are also found in those with learning disability and schizophrenia. However, it may sometimes be difficult to establish whether these have always been present and are developmental and part of the learning disability itself or whether such symptoms have arisen at a later stage in life, i.e. around adolescence. The person with learning disability may not be able to report on this, thus making it vital to obtain information from an informant, preferably a parent, who has known the person from childhood.

Another interesting twist in this context is the differential diagnosis of schizophrenia and learning disability itself. Kay (1989) comments that like people with learning disability, 'psychotics' often exhibit failures in adaptive functioning due to psychiatric rather than developmental reasons. Hence, Kay asserts that the cognitive impairment of schizophrenia can be highly similar to that of learning disability both in its quality and severity. Adding to this complexity, Kay declares that people with learning disability often resemble psychotics both in their intellectual level and behavioural profile. This confusion in differential diagnosis of learning disability and psychosis clearly calls for identifiable objective methods for differential diagnosis.

Dementia

One of the most important gains resulting from the social and economic development of the UK in the twentieth century has been the longevity of its citizens (Walker and Walker 1995). Alzheimer's disease is the most common cause of dementia and accounts for most of the irreversible dementia seen in the general population (Gregg 1994). As age is the strongest risk factor for developing dementia, the likelihood of individuals with learning disability developing dementia is also increasing. It is widely known that people with Down's syndrome can develop Alzheimer's disease by the age of 40, although many do not demonstrate the clinical features of dementia (Oliver and Holland 1986; Tuinier and Verhoeven 1993). There are reports of high prevalence rates of dementia in people with Down's syndrome and the rapid decline of general functioning abilities with age in this population (Tuinier and Verhoeven 1993).

Dementia is characterised by a deterioration and disintegration in the intellectual, affective and behavioural aspect of an individual. It is nearly always progressive and occurs in the setting of clear consciousness (Reid 1985). The symptoms of dementia in adults with Down's syndrome are diverse, encompassing both personality changes and cognitive decline. These include seizures, loss of speech, disorientation, excessive concern regarding health, disorientation, stereotyped behaviour, impaired learning, loss of vocational skills, fine tremors of fingers and intellectual deterioration (Burt et al. 1992; Aylward et al. 1995; Sung et al. 1997).

Although current diagnostic systems encompass learning disability and dementia, they do not address the issue of the impact of dementia in adults with learning disability. Hence, the American Association on Mental Retardation (AAMR) and the International Association for the Scientific Study of Intellectual Disability (IASSID) jointly formed a working group for the establishment of the criteria for the diagnosis of dementia in people with learning disability (Aylward et al. 1995). This report attempts to provide criteria based on ICD-10, by highlighting issues concerned with memory decline, decline in other cognitive functions, awareness of environment, emotional control, motivation and social behaviour. The story of James highlights some of the behaviours associated with dementia.

> James is a 51-year-old man with Downs's syndrome. His GP referred him to a psychiatric clinic in the belief that he might be suffering from early dementia. Thyroid function tests and routine blood tests, including blood sugar, were reported as being normal.
>
> Reports from carers and baseline assessment showed good vision and hearing. James is able to understand simple conversations and communicate basic needs. There are no mobility problems. He can dress without physical assistance. He is able to feed himself with a knife and fork but tends to be messy. He understands the concept of time, that is, he can tell morning from afternoon. James has a poor concept of money and poor literacy skills. He was not showing any behavioural changes.

James lives in a supported tenancy. He has become increasingly forgetful over the last 6 months, for example he would go to the bathroom with a towel for a shower and forget why he had gone there. He has started getting lost in town, whereas previously he knew where shops were; he now requires supervision when going out. James has a good memory for past events but poor recent memory. He is waking up earlier, e.g. at 5.00 a.m. There is no change in his interest or enjoyment of activities or in appetite; he has not suffered weight loss. He is not tearful and there have been no recorded seizures. James moved to his present accommodation some years ago and coped well with the change. He attends a day centre 5 days a week.

According to ICD-10 diagnostic guidelines, dementia is a syndrome due to disease of the brain, usually of a chronic or progressive nature, in which there is disturbance of multiple higher cortical functions, including memory, thinking, orientation, comprehension, calculation, learning capacity, language and judgement. Consciousness is not clouded. Impairments of cognitive function are commonly accompanied, and occasionally preceded, by deterioration in emotional control, social behaviour or motivation. This syndrome occurs in Alzheimer's disease, in cerebrovascular disease and in other conditions primarily or secondarily affecting the brain.

Dementia produces an appreciable decline in intellectual functioning, and usually some interference with personal activities of daily living, such as washing, dressing, eating, personal hygiene, excretory and toilet activities. How such a decline manifests itself will depend largely on the social and cultural setting in which the patient lives.

Diagnostic issues of dementia in learning disabilities

In the diagnosis and care of people with learning disability and dementia, the non-cognitive symptoms that occur as part of the dementing process are of additional importance. Indeed, Cooper and Prasher (1998) suggest that such symptoms are a common feature of dementia in people with Down's syndrome and in people with learning disability of other aetiologies.

The diagnosis of Alzheimer's disease and dementia in people with Down's syndrome and in other people with learning disability is of critical importance in providing appropriate care and intervention for this client group. Zigman et al. (1996) suggest that there is an increased risk of dementia among adults with Down's syndrome over 50 years of age and this provides strong evidence that current neuropathological criteria for diagnosis of Alzheimer's disease are not strongly related to clinical expression of symptoms. Therefore, the use of multiple outcome measures with varying diagnostic criteria can provide reliable estimates of the differences in risk of dementia.

The co-occurrence of dementia and depression in people with learning disabilities has also been reported (Lai 1992). People with Down's syndrome who are also severely depressed are more likely to develop dementia compared with those individuals who experience moderate depression (Burt et al. 1992; Reiss and Benson 1985). As dementia can have both direct and indirect consequences on aspects of daily functioning, this could distort the diagnosis of depression. In addition to these issues, people with Down's syndrome are prone to medical conditions, such as hypothyroidism, which cause depression.

The occurrence of depression and dementia and the difficulty of differential diagnosis emphasise the need for practitioners to investigate several different areas. In order to determine patterns of change in a person's life, areas such as social support, expressive language, social skills, daily living skills, developmental or life changes and potential life stresses need to be examined (Sung et al. 1997). It is further reported that a multidimensional analysis of qualitative and quantitative measures of daily functioning across an extended period of time can help to unravel the complexities surrounding this problem, which affect a growing number of ageing adults with Down's syndrome. Hence, the main issue in this context rests on dementia's appropriate diagnosis and care. Although there is good awareness that people with Down's syndrome are at increased risk of developing dementia at a younger age, there is less emphasis on dementia occurring in older people with learning disabilities of other causes.

Personality disorders

Personality disorders are defined in DSM-IV-TR as an enduring pattern of inner experience and behaviour that deviates markedly from the expectations of the individual's culture and is pervasive and inflexible, has an onset that can be traced back to at least adolescence or early adulthood, is stable over time and leads to distress or impairment. It further states that this enduring pattern is manifested in two or more of the following areas:

(1) Cognition – ways of perceiving and interpreting self, other people and events
(2) Affectivity – the range, intensity, lability and appropriateness of emotional response
(3) Interpersonal functioning
(4) Impulse control

DSM-IV-TR further states that this pattern should be stable and of long duration, should not be better accounted for by another mental disorder and should not be directly related to the effects of a substance, for example a drug of abuse or medication, or a general medical condition, for example a head injury.

DSM-IV-TR defines mental retardation as significantly subaverage intellectual functioning (IQ of 70 or below) with concurrent deficits in adaptive functioning, that is, the person's effectiveness in meeting the expectations of his or her culture in areas of communication, self-care, home living, social/interpersonal skills, use of community resources, self-direction, functional academic skills, work, leisure, health and safety. The onset should be before age 18.

Looking at the above definitions of personality disorder and mental retardation one can see that both are developmental disorders with onset before adulthood and are long lasting. People with mental retardation as defined are likely to have impairment of cognition due to their intellectual deficits, problems with impulsivity and mood lability due to brain dysfunction and associated less effective internal controls, and experience social consequences of their disability, with difficulties in establishing trusting relationships due to their dependence on others for basic needs, care and protection. Thus one can see that there is a considerable overlap between the definitions of personality disorder and mental retardation, which makes the diagnosis of personality disorder particularly difficult in those with learning disability.

The other difficulty in diagnosis is defining in a person with learning disability the age range within which normal adolescence occurs. This is the time when a lasting sense of self (personal identity) is established. During this stage young people start striving to become more independent by trying out new things that their parents may not necessarily approve of or expressing personal views that may be different from their parents' views. In an ordinary person, lasting personality characteristics that define the person as an adult are noticeable by adolescence or early adulthood. With people with learning disability, due to their dependency needs, parents and carers are likely to find it more difficult to 'let go' in the same way as parents of ordinary adolescents can. People with severe or profound learning disability are likely to find it difficult to establish any form of 'real' independence from their parents or carers, given that they are functioning at a mental age of less than 3 years. Thus it is possible that the development of self-identity could be a life-long process. It is estimated that even a person functioning in the mild learning disability range (IQ 50 to 69) has a mental age of between 9 to 12.

Formal efforts to describe abnormal personality traits began in the early nineteenth century as European psychiatrists Pinel and Esquirol Pritchard and the American psychiatrist Rush described persons whose behaviour violated social norms. Such persons would now be regarded as having antisocial personality disorders. In the early twentieth century Freud and Janet described psychological traits associated with hysteria, now called histrionic personality disorder. The current classification system DSM-IV-TR lists ten personality disorders grouped in three clusters. Cluster A includes the so-called eccentric group – paranoid, schizoid and schizotypal personality disorders. Cluster B includes the 'dramatic' disorders – antisocial, borderline, histrionic and narcissistic personality disorders. These are characterised by a pervasive pattern of violating social norms (for example criminal behaviour, impulsivity, excessive emotionality, grandiosity) or 'acting out' (examples include tantrums, self-abusive behaviour and anger outbursts). Cluster C consists of the 'anxious' disorders – avoidant, dependent and obsessive–compulsive personality disorders. From the above classifications one can see that people with learning disability are more likely to fall into cluster B and C groups due to their developmental issues rather than necessarily a mental disorder called personality disorder. Furthermore the DSM-IV-TR multi-axial system of classification groups both personality disorders and mental retardation in axis II to distinguish them from axis I disorders, such as schizophrenia and other psychotic disorders, mood disorders, i.e. depressive and bipolar disorders, anxiety disorders and organic brain disorders such as dementias and delirium or substance-related disorders (American Psychiatric Association 2000).

Thus personality disorders are characterised by maladaptive patterns of behaviour. Menolascino and Potter (1989) state that personality disorders are qualitatively different from psychotic or anxiety disorders, but in what form they differ is not made explicit in the literature. As personality disorders are more concerned with maladaptive patterns of behaviour, there is the possibility of overclassifying some of the behavioural symptoms as personality disorder. There is evidence to suggest this has happened, as among first admissions of people with learning disability to hospitals, personality disorder constituted the most common diagnosis (Day 1985). The story of Alan helps us to understand the nature of personality disorder in a young person with learning disabilities.

Alan is a 25-year-old with mild learning disabilities. He has a long history of anti-social behaviour, consisting of physical assaults and inappropriate sexual behaviour. Alan requires encouragement and prompts to complete tasks, for example personal hygiene, keeping his room tidy, doing his laundry, etc. He has difficulties in interacting with others and makes inappropriate personal remarks of an insulting nature to people whom he does not know; thus he frequently gets into conflict with other people. He suffers from mood swings, consisting of episodes of extreme aggression and verbal abuse, with threatening behaviour.

His personality assessment indicates features of avoidant, anti-social and schizoid personality traits. He has, in the past, made attempts to harm himself by cutting his forearm superficially. He has disclosed sexual interest in children to a number of people on separate occasions.

Alan has had a difficult, traumatic upbringing. His parents divorced when he was young and his mother had several partners afterwards. Many of these partners were physically abusive to both his mother and himself, so he experienced chaotic upbringing with little stability or exposure to positive male role models. He has a long history of behavioural difficulties from childhood. This developed into offending behaviours in adolescence and adulthood. Alan has a tendency to abuse alcohol but denies illicit drug use. As a child, Alan was said to be hyperactive with poor impulse control. He frequently fought with other children at school. He could not settle into normal school and hence went to special school from the age of 6. He frequently truanted from school. He was taken into local authority care at age 15.

Alan has a past history of deliberate self-harm, including taking an overdose. Reports suggest that he does not always tell the truth. Diagnosis: dissocial personality disorder, ICD-10, in addition to mild learning disabilities.

ICD-10 notes that personality disorders are 'developmental conditions which appear in late childhood or adolescence and continue into adulthood'. Furthermore 'they are not secondary to another mental disorder or to brain disease, although they may precede or coexist with other disorders'. In contrast, 'personality change is acquired during adult life, following severe or prolonged stress, extreme environmental deprivation, serious psychiatric disorder or brain disease or injury'. Personality disorders according to ICD-10 represent extreme or significant deviations from the way in which the average individual in a given culture perceives, thinks, feels and, particularly, relates to others. Can we define an average individual within the learning disability spectrum? If we are unable to define such an individual then the boundaries between normality and disorder become blurred, with the potential for overdiagnosis, inappropriate labelling and stigmatising individuals who may be actually functioning and behaving like the majority of their peers within a given range of learning disability.

Personality disorders represent a severe disturbance in the characterological constitution and behavioural tendencies of the individual, usually involving several areas of the personality, and nearly always associated with considerable personal and social disruption. Personality disorder tends to appear in late childhood or adolescence and continues to be manifest into adulthood. It is therefore unlikely that the diagnosis of personality disorder will be appropriate before the age of 16 or 17. General diagnostic guidelines applying to all personality disorders are presented below; supplementary descriptions are provided with each of the subtypes.

Diagnostic guidelines for personality disorders

The following is a list of criteria for personality disorders not directly attributable to gross brain damage or disease or to another psychiatric disorder:

(1)   Markedly disharmonious attitudes and behaviour are exhibited, involving usually several areas of functioning, such as affectivity, arousal, impulse control, ways of perceiving and thinking, and style of relating to others.
(2)   The abnormal behaviour pattern is enduring, long standing and not limited to episodes of mental illness.
(3)   The abnormal behaviour pattern is pervasive and clearly maladaptive to a broad range of personal and social situations.
(4)   The above manifestations always appear during childhood or adolescence and continue into adulthood.
(5)   The disorder leads to considerable personal distress, but this may only become apparent late in its course.

(6) The disorder is usually, but not invariably, associated with significant problems in occupational and social performance.

Diagnostic issues of personality disorders in learning disabilities

The low incidence of personality disorder in the community could be attributed to its underdiagnosis in this population because the diagnosis of better known mental health disorders takes precedence and co-existing personality disorders may be ignored (Khan et al. 1997). In the assessment and diagnosis of personality disorder, it is vital that the psychiatric assessments distinguish between long-standing personality abnormalities stemming from early adolescence and psychiatric and behavioural problems arising in later life. Khan et al. (1997), in their survey of personality disorders in people with learning disability, found that mainly impulsive and anti-social types were referred to psychiatrists.

In a recent review of the diagnosis of personality disorders in learning disability, Alexander and Cooray (2003) found that the prevalence ranged from less than 1 to 91% in community settings and 22 to 92% in hospital settings. These differences in prevalence were too large to be explained by real differences. They conclude that the diagnosis of personality disorders in this group is complex and difficult, particularly in those with severe disability. They recommend that developing consensus diagnostic criteria specific for various developmental levels with inclusion of proxy measures such as behavioural observations and informant accounts may be one way forward in the future.

Multiple diagnostic presentations and differential diagnosis

In addition to the diagnosis of learning disability, some individuals have a number of neurological, chromosomal and genetic abnormalities that contribute to the nature of manifestation of mental health disorders. The simultaneous occurrence of challenging behaviour and mental health disorders in this population may indicate some association between them. There is evidence to suggest that some form of self-injurious behaviour may be associated with obsessive–compulsive disorder (Bodfish et al. 1995) and that fluctuations in mood state associated with affective disorders may provide the motivational basis for other forms of self-injury (Sovner and Pary 1993). There is also evidence suggesting an association between challenging behaviour and depression. Meins (1995) reports that people who find it difficult to express their emotions verbally may exhibit aggressive behaviour, withdrawal and somatic complaints instead of classic depressive complaints such as feelings of hopelessness.

The diagnosis of mental health disorders in people with learning disability is a complex process due to the multiple presentations of symptoms. For example, while diagnosing affective disorders, it is important that clinicians should take note of drug-induced depression. Van Putten and May (1978) comment that antipsychotic drug-induced akinesia, a type of Parkinsonian reaction, can be misdiagnosed as depression. It is suggested that extrapyramidal side effects are associated with a reduced range of facial expression, psycho-motor retardation and apathy (Sovner and Pary 1993), and hence this could be confused with depression. There are also reports of simultaneous presenta-tions of epilepsy and mental health disorders. Crawford (1997) warns that if a person with learning disabilities has sudden episodes of 'depression' lasting a few days or weeks combined with incontinence and refusal to eat, it may indicate signs of epilepsy and an electroencephalogram might be useful for differential diagnosis.

It is also possible that schizophrenic symptoms may co-exist with the features of mania to produce the mixed clinical picture referred to as schizo-affective disorders (Lyttle 1985). As opposed to major depression and bipolar disorder with psychotic features, the psychotic component of this disorder may be manifested not only in the presence of affective symptoms, but also independ-ently. In order to meet the diagnostic criteria of schizo-affective illness, it is suggested that the individual must meet the criteria for schizophrenia as well as that for an affective disorder (Sovner and Pary 1993). To aid the differential diagnosis, Levitt and Tsuang (1988) suggest that it is important to differentiate between the bipolar form which may be a variant of typical bipolar illness and the depressive type which may be more closely related to schizophrenia. It is interesting to note that there is very little evidence of schizo-affective dis-orders in people with learning disabilities. Tyrer and Dunstan (1997) point out that the lack of reports of schizo-affective disorders in people with learning disabilities may suggest that it is only very rarely exhibited.

There are also issues concerning the presentation of autistic spectrum dis-orders. Autism is a syndrome of multiple aetiologies, and several disease entities – genetic, metabolic and structural – are associated with it (Read 1997). This includes infantile hydrocephalus, tuberous sclerosis and fragile X syn-drome. It is possible for the autistic disorder to be confused with schizophrenia; however, as people with autistic spectrum disorders do not exhibit or describe hallucinations or delusions, this helps with the differential diagnosis (Tyrer and Dunstan 1997).

One of the commonly observed medical conditions among people with Down's syndrome is hypothyroidism. An underactive thyroid can lead to progressive loss of interest and initiative, slowing of mental processes, poor memory for recent events, fading of the personality's colour and vivacity, general intellec-tual deterioration, depression with a paranoid flavour, and eventually, if not checked, to dementia and permanent harmful effects on the brain (Awad 1986). As the thyroid problem often develops insidiously over a considerable period of time, it is possible that this may not be adequately detected in people with Down's syndrome and this could be confused with depressive disorders or dementia.

Psychiatric assessment in routine clinical practice

A clinician assessing a patient for a possible mental disorder needs to collect clinical data objectively and accurately by history taking and examination of the mental state and organise these data in a systematic way. The hierarchical multi-axial classification systems of ICD-10 and DC-LD are particularly helpful here for adults with learning disabilities. A clinician also needs to have an intuitive understanding of the patient as an individual based on their previous life experiences.

The assessment needs to provide enough information to decide whether there is a disorder and if so what kind of disorder, and to formulate a care plan to help the patient and his/her carers. A comprehensive appraisal usually requires assessment by a multidisciplinary team, and the role of the psychiatrist is in helping to develop a comprehensive biopsychosocial formulation of the presenting problem and devising a comprehensive and holistic treatment plan based on the formulation. Learning disability nurses play a significant role here in coordinating, planning and conducting the assessment process, using assessment schedules such as mini PAS-ADD (Psychiatric Assessment Schedule for Adults with Developmental Disability), tailor-made observation charts of daily behaviour and observation of the side effects of medication.

Information is obtained from the patient and informants who know the person well. It is important to choose informants who have known the person well for an adequate length of time and with whom they spend regular time. Information from informants in different settings, for example the day centre or college, may be required. In this context parents are able to provide detailed information about the person's early development, adverse experiences, and the person's skills and temperament before the onset of the disorder.

It is important to separate symptoms of disorder and their consequences from the impairment, disability and handicap associated with the learning disability itself. Impairment refers to the interference with the functioning of a psychological or physical system such as memory, mood regulation, attention and concentration. Disability refers to the interference with the activities of the whole person, for example inability to dress or feed oneself, walk independently and so on. Handicap refers to the social disadvantage resulting from the impairment and disability, for example inability to work or fulfil roles expected of the person as an adult, e.g. that of spouse or parent (Gelder et al. 2001). Note that the mental disorder will also be associated with impairment, disability and handicap, which may be further compounded by the pre-existing deficits associated with the learning disability itself. An additional mental illness such as schizophrenia may result in further impairment of both intelligence and social or adaptive functioning which may be difficult to define clearly unless one has good collateral information about the person's level of functioning before the onset of the illness process.

Information and history-taking for assessment and diagnosis

Traditionally information collected from a patient is categorised as follows:

(1) Name, age and address of patient; name of informant(s) and their relationship to patient, how long they have known the patient and how much time they spend with them on a weekly basis.
(2) Reason for the referral.
(3) History of the present illness.
(4) Family history: mental disorder or learning disability among parents or siblings may indicate genetic or environmental influences. The personalities and attitudes of parents or carers are important in understanding the environmental context in which the person grew up. Marital disharmony, separation, divorce, remarriage, how the family coped with having a child with learning disability, the material circumstances, occupation of the parents and how siblings coped with their disabled brother or sister are areas that can be explored further. Recent bereavements, serious illness or other stressful events, for example having to move into care after death of last surviving parent, may all be relevant to explore further.
(5) Personal history:
   — Pregnancy and birth: prolonged labour, difficult birth, forceps delivery, breathing difficulties at birth and prematurity are some of the areas to explore here.
   — Early development: feeding difficulty as infant, when milestones were attained, for example sitting up, walking, babbling, speaking in sentences, becoming dry during day time, age when dry both ways, i.e. continent of faeces and urine. Recurrence of bed wetting may be an important clue to a stressful event during childhood. Separation from primary caregiver for any reason may be important.
   — Health in childhood: minor childhood ailments, epilepsy, asthma, repeated chest or ear infections, etc.
   — Education: whether statemented under the Education Act, mainstream or special schooling, additional support in mainstream school, relationships with peers, whether bullied or called names, and quality of teaching may all be relevant here. Include details of any higher education.
   — Work history.
   — Relationships, including sexual experience if any.
   — Social circumstances.
   — Substance use: abuse of alcohol as a way of coping with anxiety and insecurity, or use of illegal substances under the influence of peers in order to feel accepted or to belong.
   — Premorbid personality: self-confidence, character (for example whether shy, introverted or extrovert, generally cheerful, moody, or irritable), strengths, moral values, weaknesses, e.g. if easily led or unable to protect self from abuse or exploitation, may all be areas to explore here.

(6) Mental state examination:
   — Appearance and behaviour.
   — Mood: depressed, anxious, high, irritable, suspicious. Whether mood is unduly labile or incongruous to the circumstances. Is there reduced emotional expression or flat affect?
   — Speech: spontaneous, coherent, relevant. Is there pressure of speech (speaking too fast) or is it too slow, lacks spontaneity and is mono-syllabic? Is there dysarthria (making speech difficult to understand) or dysphasia (disorder of fluency, intonation) etc?
   — Thought: form and content, for example is the thought content dis-organised and difficult to follow or illogical? Is there poverty of thought (few thoughts) or pressure of thoughts (too many thoughts)? Is the normal boundary of the thought processes maintained, i.e. thought being private to oneself and confined to one's mind? Are there obsessional ruminations or compulsive rituals associated with obsessional thoughts? Are there negative cognitions, excess worrying thoughts, suicidal ideas or delusional beliefs? Are there any perceptual disturbances (for example hallucinations in different modalities, illu-sions or vivid fantasy)?
   — Attention: concentration and memory, clouding of consciousness and confusion.
   — Insight: whether the person recognises that he/she has a problem or is ill, the nature of the problem (whether it is physical or mental), possible causes, the need for treatment, and type of help available including medication and psychological treatments.
(7) Physical examination.
(8) Special investigations: chromosome analysis, DNA studies, computerised tomography or magnetic resonance imaging brain scan, electroencephalo-gram, etc.
(9) Psychological assessment: intelligence tests, neuropsychological tests, standardised behaviour rating scales, functional analysis of behavioural problems, etc.

Special considerations when assessing people with learning disabilities

Diagnosis in the general public relies mainly on the person being able to describe his or her thoughts, perceptions, feelings and life circumstances and observa-tions in clinical interview. In a person with severe learning disability where the individual can say little about his or her thoughts and feelings one has to rely more on third party information and direct observations of the person's behaviour and functioning in different settings.

A number of factors may influence the ability of the person with learning disability to communicate effectively. These include deficits due to neurolo-gical factors related to pre-existing brain damage or epilepsy or the side effects of drugs, for example excessive sedation. The mental disorder itself may further impair already limited communicative competence, for example thought disorder associated with schizophrenia, withdrawal associated with severe depression or poor memory associated with dementia. The previous experiences of the person, for example whether he or she was brought up in a positive enabling environment or in a punitive, restrictive environment, may be relevant. The severity of the learning disability will obviously have implications regarding the quantity and quality of information given through either verbal or non-verbal means. Learning disability itself may lead to limited verbal fluency, limited understanding, impaired speech production, sensory deficits (for example poor hearing or vision), behavioural disturbance and limited attention span. The individual may have had previous negative interview experiences, for example psychological testing or a hospital interview that has led to admission to a special hospital without the person having any say in what happened. Leudar and Fraser (1985) noted that communication is frequently disrupted not only by the lack of linguistic skills but also by behaviour problems, in particular communicative withdrawal. They described the 'withdrawal strategies' that some people with learning disabilities use, for example not initiating conversation, giving limited information, replying 'I don't know' or 'I can't remember' to most questions, gesturing non-co-operation by turning head away or shaking head when no question is being asked.

General guidelines for interviewing people with learning disabilities

In the case of a referral of a person with learning disabilities to psychiatric services, usually someone other than the person with the learning disability raises concern about the problem and asks for help. Often family carers or nurses rather than the person with the learning difficulty may notice a change in the person's day-to-day functioning. Changes in the tolerance of carers may result in referral of someone whose behaviour has not objectively changed or changes in carers may result in an old problem previously tolerated being referred. Changes in social environment may result in what was before a minor irritant escalating into an intolerable problem.

It is important to allow adequate time for the assessment without undue interruptions from bleeps, etc. The setting where the assessment is carried out is also an important consideration. For example the person's home, day centre or a familiar place may be more productive than the unfamiliar setting of a hospital outpatient clinic. A noise free environment is important. Thus politely asking the person or carers to turn the radio or television off and to ensure there is no interruption from other sources is helpful.

A relaxed, informal, conversational style to make the person feel at ease is vital at the beginning of the first interview. Asking the person about his or her current interests and daily familiar routines may be helpful in developing a good rapport. Knowing about important recent events, such as birthdays and holidays, can help set the presenting problems within a coherent timeframe.

It is important to explain the purpose of the interview and issues related to confidentiality. An active listening stance with frequent clarification to check that the person understands the issues is clearly helpful. Try to use jargon-free, straightforward language with short sentences. It helps to be concrete and use open questions initially to ensure that information given is spontaneous as far as possible. Rephrase questions in different ways to check understanding and ensure that the information given is reliable and consistent. Try to ask one question at a time and allow enough time for a reply. It is important to avoid unnecessary interruption. People with learning disability find questions related to 'present and concrete' events easier to answer than abstract questions about the 'future'. Questions related to time and frequency also may be more difficult. It is important to be sensitive to non-verbal signals, for example facial expressions, tone of voice, signs of agitation. Suggestibility, that is, the person saying what he/she thinks the interviewer wants to hear rather than what he/she actually thinks, is an important phenomenon to be aware of. Similarly acquiescence (saying yes to any question) could be a difficulty ('same answer' problem). Thus it is important to cross-check the information obtained at the interview with key workers, case records and previous assessments.

Conclusion

The detection and diagnosis of mental health disorders in people with learning disabilities is a complex process due to their limited vocabulary, insight and skills deficits. The assessment process should include details of their skills and abilities, nature and pattern of behaviour in a range of environments, relationships and understanding of their own emotions and of other people around them. The diagnostic criteria provide us with the objectivity to assess the symptoms of mental illness in people with learning disabilities. However, there are limitations to these due to communication difficulties and we should in the future explore and adapt appropriate ways of assessing mental health disorders in people with learning disabilities.

References

Alexander, S. and Cooray, S. (2003) Diagnosis of personality disorders in learning disability. *British Journal of Psychiatry*, **182** (44), 28–31.

Aman, M.G. et al. (1985) The aberrant behaviour checklist: a behaviour rating scale for the assessment of treatment effects. *American Journal of Mental Deficiency*, **89**, 485–491.

American Psychiatric Association (1994) *Diagnostic and Statistical Manual of Mental Disorders (DSM-IV)*. Washington DC: APA.

American Psychiatric Association (2000) *Diagnostic and Statistical Manual of Mental Disorders (DSM-IV-TR)*. Washington DC: APA.

Awad, A.G. (1986) *The Thyroid and the Mind and Emotions – Thyroid Dysfunction and Mental Health Disorders*. www.home.ican.net/~thyroid/articles/enge10f.html.

Aylward, E.H., Burt, D.B., Thorpe, L.U., Lai, F. and Dalton, A.J. (1995) *Diagnosis of Dementia in Individuals with Intellectual Disability*. Washington DC: American Association on Mental Retardation.

Bailey, N.M. and Andrews, T.M. (2003) Diagnostic criteria for psychiatric disorders for use with adults with learning disabilities/mental retardation (DC-LD) and the diagnosis of anxiety disorders: a review. *Journal of Intellectual Disability Research*, **47** (Suppl. 1), 50–61.

Ballinger, B.R., Ballinger, C.B., Reid, A.H. and McQueen, E. (1991) The psychiatric symptoms, diagnoses and care needs of 100 mentally handicapped patients. *British Journal of Psychiatry*, **158**, 255–259.

Beck, A.T., Ward, C.H., Mendelson, M., Mock, J. and Erbaugh, J. (1961) An inventory for measuring depression. *Archives of General Psychiatry*, **4**, 53–63.

Beier, A.L. (1919) Cited in Gostason, R. (1985) Psychiatric illness among the mentally retarded: a Swedish population study. *Acta Psychiatrica Scandinavica*, **71**, Suppl. 318, 23.

Bodfish, J.W., Cranford, T.W., Powell, S.B., Parker, D.E., Golden, R.N. and Lewis, M.H. (1995) Compulsions in adults with mental retardation: prevalence, phenomenology and co-morbidity with stereotypy and self-injury. *American Journal of Mental Retardation*, **100**, 183–192.

Burt, D.B., Loveland, K.A. and Lewis, K.R. (1992) Depression and the onset of dementia in adults with mental retardation. *American Journal of Mental Retardation*, **96**, 502–511.

Campbell, M. and Malone, R.P. (1991) Mental retardation and psychiatric disorders. *Hospital and Community Psychiatry*, **42**, 374–379.

Charlot, L.R., Doucette, A.C. and Mezzacappa, E. (1993) Affective symptoms of institutionalised adults with mental retardation. *American Journal of Mental Retardation*, **98** (3), 408–416.

Cooper, S.A. and Callacott, R.A. (1994) Clinical features and diagnostic criteria of depression in Down's syndrome. *British Journal of Psychiatry*, **165**, 399–403.

Cooper, S.A. and Prasher, V.P. (1998) Maladaptive behaviours and symptoms of dementia in adults with Down's syndrome compared with intellectual disability of other aetiologies. *Journal of Intellectual Disability Research*, **42**, 293–300.

Corbett, J.A. (1979) Psychiatric morbidity and mental retardation. In: F.E. James and R.P. Snaith (Eds) *Psychiatric Illness and Mental Handicap*. London: Gaskell Press.

Crawford, P. (1997) Epilepsy and learning disabilities. In: S. Read (Ed.) *Psychiatry in Learning Disability*. London: W.B. Saunders.

Cutts, R.A. (1957) Differentiation between pseudo-mental defectives with emotional disorders and mental defectives with emotional disturbances. *American Journal of Mental Deficiency*, **61**, 716–722.

Day, K. (1985) Psychiatric disorders in the middle aged and elderly mentally handicapped. *British Journal of Psychiatry*, **147**, 660–667.

DesNoyers-Hurley, A. and Silka, V.R. (2003) Identification of hallucinations and delusions in people with intellectual disability. *Mental Health Aspects of Developmental Disabilities*, **6**, 153–157.

Doody, G., Johnstone, E., Sanderson, T., Owens, D. and Muir, W. (1998) 'Propfschizophrenie' revisited. Schizophrenia in people with mild learning disability. *British Journal of Psychiatry*, **173**, 145–153.

Dosen, A. (1993) Mental health and mental illness in persons with retardation: what are we talking about? In: R. Fletcher and A. Dosen (Eds) *Mental Health Aspects of Mental Retardation*. New York: Lexington Books.

Eaton, L.F. and Menolascino, F.J. (1982) Psychiatric disorders in the mentally retarded: types, problems and challenges. *American Journal of Psychiatry*, **139**, 1297–1303.

Enfield, S.L. (1992) Clinical assessment of psychiatric symptoms in mentally retarded individuals. *Australian and New Zealand Journal of Psychiatry*, **26**, 48–63.

Enfield, S.L. and Aman, M. (1995) Issues in the taxonomy of psychopathology in mental retardation. *Journal of Autism and Developmental Disorders*, **25**, 143–167.

Febrega, H. (1994) International systems of diagnosis in psychiatry. *Journal of Nervous and Mental Disease*, **182**, 256–263.

Fraser, W.I. and Nolan, M. (1994) Psychiatric disorders in mental retardation. In: N. Bouras (Ed.) *Mental Health in Mental Retardation: Recent Advances*. Cambridge: Cambridge University Press.

Fraser, W.I., Leuder, I., Gray, J. and Campbell, I. (1986) Psychiatric and behaviour disturbance in mental handicap. *Journal of Mental Deficiency Research*, **30**, 49–57.

Gedye, A. (1992) Recognising obsessive–compulsive disorder claims in clients with developmental disabilities. *The Habilitative Mental Health Care Newsletter*, **11**, 73–74.

Gelder, M., Mayou, R. and Cowen, P. (2001) *Shorter Oxford Textbook of Psychiatry, Part 1.* Oxford: Oxford Medical Publications.

Gregg, D. (1994) *Alzheimer's Disease (Harvard Health Letter Special Report)*. Cambridge, Massachusetts: Harvard Medical School.

Hamilton, M. (1960) A rating scale for depression. *Journal of Neurology, Neurosurgery and Psychiatry*, **23**, 56–62.

Helsel, W.J. and Matson, J.L. (1988) The relationship of depression to social skills and intellectual functioning in mentally retarded adults. *Journal of Mental Deficiency Research*, **32**, 411–418.

Jacobson, J. (1990) Do some mental disorders occur less frequently among persons with mental retardation? *American Journal of Mental Retardation*, **94**, 596–602.

James, D.H., Mukherjee, T. and Smith, C. (1996) Schizophrenia and learning disability. *British Journal of Learning Disabilities*, **24**, 90–94.

Kay, S. (1989) Cognitive battery for differential diagnosis of mental retardation vs. psychosis. *Research in Developmental Disabilities*, **10**, 251–260.

Kazdin, A.E., Matson, J. and Senatore, V. (1983) Assessment of depression in the mentally retarded adults. *American Journal of Psychiatry*, **140**, 1040–1043.

Kessler, R.C., McGonagle, K.A. and Zhao, S. (1994) Lifetime and 12-month prevalence of DSM-III-R psychiatric disorders in the United States: results from the National Comorbidity Survey. *Archives of General Psychiatry*, **51**, 8–19.

Khan, A., Cowan, C. and Roy, A. (1997) Personality disorders in people with learning disabilities: a community survey. *Journal of Intellectual Disability Research*, **41**, 324–330.

Kraeplin, E. (1919) Cited in Gostason, R. (1985) Psychiatric illness among the mentally retarded: a Swedish population study. *Acta Psychiatrica Scandinavica*, **71**, Suppl. 318, 25.

Lai, F. (1992) Clinical pathological features of Alzheimer disease and Down's syndrome. In: L. Nadel and C.J. Epstein (Eds) *Down's Syndrome and Alzheimer Disease*. New York: Wiley-Liss.

Leudar, I. and Fraser, W. (1985) How to keep quiet: some withdrawal strategies in mentally handicapped adults. *Journal of Mental Deficiency Research*, **129** (4), 315–330.

Levitt, J.J. and Tsuang, M.T. (1988) The heterogeneity of schizoaffective disorder: implications for treatment. *American Journal of Psychiatry*, **145**, 926–936.

Lyttle, J. (1985) *Mental Disorder: Its Care and Treatment*. London: Baillière Tindall.

Marston, G.M., Perry, D.W. and Roy, A. (1997) Manifestation of depression in people with intellectual disability. *Journal of Intellectual Disability Research*, **41**, 476–480.

McCarthy, J. (2001) Post-traumatic stress disorder in people with learning disability. *Advances in Psychiatric Treatment*, **7**, 163–169.

McCracken, J.T. and Diamond, R.P. (1988) Bipolar disorder in mentally retarded adolescents. *Journal of the American Academy of Child and Adolescent Psychiatry*, **27**, 494–499.

Meins, W. (1995) Symptoms of major depression in mentally retarded adults. *Journal of Intellectual Disability Research*, **39**, 41–45.

Menolascino, F.J. and Potter, J.F. (1989) Mental illness in the elderly mentally retarded. *Journal of Applied Gerontology*, **8**, 192–202.

Mittler, P. (1979) *People Not Patients: Problems and Policies in Mental Handicap*. London: Methuen.

Moss, S., Prosser, H. and Goldberg, D. (1996) Validity of the schizophrenia diagnosis of the psychiatric assessment schedule for adults with developmental disability (PAS-ADD). *British Journal of Psychiatry*, **168**, 359–367.

Offord, D. and Cross, L. (1971) Adult schizophrenia with scholastic failure or low IQ in childhood. *Archives of General Psychiatry*, **24**, 431–436.

Oliver, C. and Holland, A.J. (1986) Down's syndrome and Alzheimer's disease: a review. *Psychological Medicine*, **16**, 307–322.

Ollendick, T.H. and Ollendick, D.G. (1982) Anxiety disorders. In: J.L. Matson and R.P. Barrett (Eds) *Psychopathology in the Mentally Retarded*. New York: Grune and Stratton.

Patel, P., Goldberg, D. and Moss, S. (1993) Psychiatric morbidity in older people with moderate and severe learning disability: the Prevalence Study. *British Journal of Psychiatry*, **163**, 481–491.

Raghavan, R. (1998) Anxiety disorders in people with learning disabilities: a review of literature. *Journal of Learning Disability for Nursing, Health and Social Care*, **2**, 3–9.

Read, S. (1997) Organic behaviour disorder. In: S. Read (Ed.) *Psychiatry in Learning Disability*. London: W.B. Saunders.

Reid, A.H. (1972) Psychoses in adult mental defectives: I. Manic depressive psychosis. *British Journal of Psychiatry*, **120**, 205–212.

Reid, A.H. (1985) Psychiatry and mental handicap. In: M. Craft, J. Bicknell and S. Hollins (Eds) *Mental Handicap: A Multidisciplinary Approach*. East Sussex: Baillière Tindall.

Reid, A.H. (1989) Psychiatry and mental handicap: a historical perspective. *Journal of Mental Deficiency Research*, **33**, 363–368.

Reiss, S. (1988) *The Reiss Screen for Maladaptive Behaviour*. Ohio: IDS Publishing.

Reiss, S. (1993) Assessment of psychopathology in persons with mental retardation. In: J.L. Matson and R.P. Barrett (Eds) *Psychopathology in the Mentally Retarded*, 2nd edition. Boston: Allyn and Bacan.

Reiss, S. and Benson, B. (1985) Psychosocial correlates of depression. *American Journal of Mental Deficiency*, **89**, 331–337.

Reiss, S., Levitan, G.W. and Szyszo, J. (1982) Emotional disturbance and mental retardation: diagnostic overshadowing. *American Journal of Mental Deficiency*, **86**, 567–574.

Royal College of Psychiatrists (2001) *DC-LD (Diagnostic Criteria for Psychiatric Disorders for Use with Adults with Learning Disabilities/Mental Retardation)*. Occasional paper OP 48. London: Gaskell Press.

Rutter, M. and Graham, P. (1970) Epidemiology of psychiatric disorder. In: M. Rutter, J. Tizard and K. Whitmore (Eds) *Education, Health, and Behaviour*. London: Longman.

Ryan, R. (1994) Post-traumatic stress disorder in persons with developmental disabilities. *Community Mental Health Journal*, **30**, 45–53.

Singh, N.N., Sood, A., Sonenklar, N. and Ellis, C. (1991) Assessment and diagnosis of mental illness in persons with mental retardation: methods and measures. *Behaviour Modification*, **15**, 419–443.

Smiley, E. and Cooper, S.A. (2003) Intellectual disabilities, depressive episode, and diagnostic criteria for psychiatric disorders for use with adults with learning disabilities/mental retardation (DC-LD). *Journal of Intellectual Disability Research*, **47** (Suppl. 1), 62–71.

Sovner, R. and DesNoyers-Hurley, A. (1986) Four factors affecting the diagnosis of psychiatric disorders in mentally retarded persons. *Psychiatric Aspects of Mental Retardation Review*, **5**, 9.

Sovner, R. and Pary, R.J. (1993) Affective disorders in developmentally disabled persons. In: J.L. Matson and R.P. Barrett (Eds) *Psychopathology in the Mentally Retarded*. Boston: Allyn and Bacan.

Spengler, P.M., Strohmer, D.C. and Prout, H.T. (1990) Testing the robustness of the diagnostic overshadowing bias. *American Journal of Mental Retardation*, **95**, 204–214.

Sturmey, P. (1995) DSM-III-R and persons with dual diagnoses: conceptual issues and strategies for future research. *Journal of Intellectual Disability Research*, **39**, 357–364.

Sturmey, P., Reed, J. and Corbett, J. (1991) Psychometric assessment of psychiatric disorders in people with learning difficulties (mental handicap): a review of measures. *Psychological Medicine*, **21**, 143–155.

Sung, H., Hawkins, B.A., Eklund, S.J., et al. (1997) Depression and dementia in ageing adults with Down's syndrome: a case study approach. *Mental Retardation*, **35**, 27–38.

Synder, S.H. (1988) *The New Biology of Mood*. New York: Pfizer.

Tomb, D. (1992) *Psychiatry*. Maryland: Williams and Wilkins.

Tuinier, S. and Verhoeven, W.M.A. (1993) Psychiatry and mental retardation: towards a behavioural pharmacological concept. *Journal of Intellectual Disability Research*, **37**, 16–25.

Turner, T.H. (1989) Schizophrenia and mental handicap: an historical review, with implications for further research. *Psychological Medicine*, **19**, 301–314.

Tyrer, S.P. and Dunstan, J.A. (1997) Schizophrenia. In: S. Read (Ed.) *Psychiatry in Learning Disability*. London: W.B. Saunders.

Van Putten, T. and May, R.P.A. (1978) 'Akinetic depression' in schizophrenia. *Archives in General Psychiatry*, **35**, 1101–1107.

Vitello, B. and Behar, D. (1992) Mental retardation and psychiatric illness. *Hospital and Community Psychiatry*, **43**, 494–499.

Walker, A. and Walker, C. (1995) Older people with learning difficulties – a new problem for the health and social services. *Paper presented at the 5th Asia/Oceanic Regional Congress of Gerontology*, Hong Kong, 19–23 November.

Weisblatt, S.A. (1994) Diagnosis of psychiatric disorders in persons with mental retardation. In: N. Bouras (Ed.) *Mental Health in Mental Retardation: Recent Advances and Practices*. Cambridge: Cambridge University Press.

White, M.J., Nichols, C.N., Cook, R.S., Spengler, P.M., Walker, B.S. and Look, K.K. (1995) Diagnostic overshadowing and mental retardation: a meta-analysis. *American Journal of Mental Retardation*, **100**, 293–298.

World Health Organization (1993) *The ICD-10 Classification of Mental and Behavioural Disorders. Diagnostic Criteria for Research*. Geneva: WHO.

Yappa, P. and Roy, A. (1990) Depressive illness and mental handicap: two case reports. *Mental Handicap*, **18**, 19–21.

Zigman, W.B., Schupf, N., Sersen, E. and Silverman, W. (1996) Prevalence of dementia in adults with and without Down's syndrome. *American Journal of Mental Retardation*, **100**, 403–412.

Zimmerman, M., Coryell, C., Corenthall, C. and Wilson, S. (1986) The research diagnostic criteria for endogenous depression and the dexomethodene suppression test: a discriminant function analysis. *Psychiatric Research*, **14**, 197–208.

Zung, W.W.K. (1965) A self-rating depression scale. *Archives of General Psychiatry*, **12**, 63–70.

Further reading

Andreasen, N.C. and Black, D.W. (2001) *Introductory Textbook of Psychiatry*, 3rd edition. Washington DC: American Psychiatric Publishing.

Cookson, J., Taylor, D. and Katona, C. (2002) *Use of Drugs in Psychiatry*, 5th edition. London: Gaskell Press.

Matson, J.L. (1988) *The PIMRA Manual*. Orland Park, Los Angeles: International Diagnostic Systems.

Matson, J., Smiroldo, B., Hamilton, M. and Bagilo, C. (1997) Do anxiety disorders exist in persons with severe and profound mental retardation? *Research in developmental disabilities*, **1**, 39–44.

Meins, W. (1993) Prevalence and risk factors for depressive disorders in adults with intellectual disability. *Australia and New Zealand Journal of Developmental Disabilities*, **18**, 147–156.

Moss, S., Prosser, H., Costello, H., et al. (1998) Reliability and validity of the PAS-ADD checklist for detecting psychiatric disorders in adults with intellectual disability. *Journal of Intellectual Disability Research*, **42** (2), 173–183.

Prosser, H., Moss, S., Costello, H., Simpson, N., Patel, P. and Rowe, S. (1998) Reliability and validity of the Mini PAS-ADD for assessing psychiatric disorders in adults with intellectual disability. *Journal of Intellectual Disability Research*, **42**, 264–272.

Chapter 5
Needs assessment

Need and *needs assessment* continue to be strong buzz words in health and social care. It is essential for professionals and service providers to understand the individual needs of service users in order to plan and provide needs-led services. The strategic planning and commissioning of services also relies on information on the population needs of a locality or community. This chapter explores the concept of need and its assessment in the context of community care for people with learning disabilities and mental illness by focusing on the development of the needs assessment schedule.

Key themes

- The concept of need and models of needs assessment
- The development of CANDID (the Camberwell Assessment of Needs for adults with Developmental and Intellectual Disability) and LDCNS (the Learning Disability version of the Cardinal Needs Schedule)
- The use of CANDID and LDCNS in identifying mental health needs and in care planning
- The role of care planning and care management using needs assessment

Introduction

The implementation of the NHS and Community Care Act 1990 (Department of Health 1990) has in many ways revolutionised the nature and pattern of care delivery for people with learning disabilities. As a result of community care, local authorities have a duty to 'assess people's needs holistically in relation to a wide range of possible service options, rather than having separate service-led assessments' (Department of Health 1991a, p. 4). The introduction of needs-based assessment is intended to mark a radical departure from previous assessment practices (Richards 1994). This is a major shift in the focus of delivery of services; people are no longer to be fitted into existing services, but services should be built around individualised needs.

The term needs assessment has been part of learning disability services since the publication of the 1971 White Paper *Better Services for the Mentally Handicapped* (Department of Health and Social Security 1971), which specified the assessment of the biopsychosocial needs of this population, in order to make statements about future services. The White Paper *Valuing People* (Department of Health 2001) refocuses on needs assessment and person-centred planning in outlining the vision of services for people with leaning disabilities. The 1971 White Paper recommended that people with learning disabilities should have equal access to the general health and social services available to everyone else.

Three decades later, the arguments and counter arguments about fully pledged ordinary mental health services for people with dual diagnosis and equal access to them are still continuing. The Reed report (Department of Health 1994) suggests that the assessment of need should be a regular joint activity, keeping the whole range of services for 'difficult to place' individuals and offender patients under review. Indeed, this process should undoubtedly enhance a planned co-ordinated service between health care services, social services and the criminal justice agencies.

Needs and needs assessment

The Department of Health document *Caring for People: Community Care in the Next Decade and Beyond* (Department of Health 1989) suggests that one of the most important aims of community care reforms is that the provision of services should be designed to suit individual needs and preferences. The proper assessment of need and good care or case management were seen as the cornerstones of the new way forward for caring for people with learning disabilities.

The Department of Health in its drive to have a common understanding of the term 'need' defines it as 'a shorthand for the requirements of individuals to enable them to achieve, maintain or restore an acceptable level of social independence or quality of life, as defined by the particular care agency or authority' (Department of Health 1991b, p. 12). It goes on to state that 'need is a dynamic concept, the definition of which will vary over time in accordance with changes in national legislation, changes in local policy, the availability of resources and the patterns of local demand'. The Department of Health in its constricted view of needs concludes that it is a relative concept and should be defined at the local level. In the context of community care and care management this entrusts the responsibility of assessing needs to local service providers.

However, the process of defining need within community care assessments is far from objective and is informed by the number of agendas, which determine the type of problems identified as well as the solutions offered. In order to bring about the paradigm shift in attitudes required on the part of professionals, it is argued that the process of defining need must become more explicit (Sim et al. 1998). In this context, Stevens and Gabbay (1991) offered a working definition of need, 'as the ability to benefit in some way from health care' (p. 21). For people with learning disability and mental health disorder, it is appropriate to amend this definition by including 'health and social care', as both these aspects are important in the context of 'ordinary life' in the community. The complexity of defining and assessing needs has been debated for many years both from a philosophical and a consumerist perspective.

The concept of need

The concept of human need has long been understood philosophically as anything that is definitionally or causally necessary for the existence of any human condition, or for the achievement of any human goal (Campbell 1974). Here, need is considered to be an abstract and an operational concept. In the abstract sense, Campbell argues that the idea of a need is almost indefinitely elastic because of the wide range of possible human conditions and purposes. However, the operational definition of need has been poorly specified or completely absent, although some attempts have been made to identify different types of need.

From a biological perspective, need is considered as a tension or a disequilibrium in the organism (Liss 1998). Liss describes how a living organism strives to keep itself in balance by struggling to maintain homeostasis. During this process, the organism is trying to maintain a balance between internal and external stimuli, thereby leading to tension. Liss argues that this disequilibrium triggers off behaviours designed to obtain objects that will lead to the reduction or elimination of tension. This results in a need and when this is satisfied the tension is eliminated.

Historically, Murray (1938) offered a list of 'needs' to account for goal seeking and motivation in human behaviour. He identified needs associated with inanimate objects, expression of ambition, power, injury to self or others, affection and other social goals. In a similar but at a higher level of human behaviour and motivation, Maslow (1954) portrayed a hierarchy of human needs based on the following dimensions of human motivation: physiology, safety, love, esteem and self-actualisation. Many aspects of care and therapy are based on Maslow's hierarchy in order to meet patient needs. Some of Maslow's expressions can be interpreted in such a way that he believes that food, security, belonging, etc. are needed in order to maintain health. Maslow (1970) believed that basic needs are human goals that 'are not only wanted and desired by all human beings, but also needed in the sense that they are necessary to avoid illness and psychopathology' (p. 13).

The teleological concept of need

Liss (1998) considers need as something instrumental or teleological because the fact that there is a need, and what there is a need for, are related to a certain goal. For example, there is a need for food, in order to survive, and there is a need for love, in order to live a satisfying and fulfilled life.

Liss suggests that when a certain thing is necessary for realising a goal it implies that this thing is lacking, and there is a deficiency of some kind. In other words, there is a *gap* between *'what is'* and *'what should be'*. Let us assume a situation where John has a need for a wheelchair. This is relevant when John lacks the wheelchair and the wheelchair is necessary in order for John to live a fulfilling life.

Liss proposes that the term *need* can be used to refer to two different things: either to a tension in the organism or to the lack of a situation (or a gap) related to a goal. He argues that the two views might in certain circumstances coincide. For example, a person suffering from shortage of body fluid and feeling thirsty might be said to have both a tension need and a teleological need for water. However, the two views of need are fundamentally different. According to Liss, to assess human need in accordance with the tension view is to register what people actually strive for. To assess human need in accordance with the teleological view is to assess what things are necessary in order to realise a certain goal (the goal could be a decent life).

In the view of need as being something goal related, X is needed when X is necessary in order to realise a goal (Wiggins 1987), and here the goal component of need is an important concept. According to Liss, the goal determines the object of need (that is, the thing needed). Hence, for example, the goal to 'live as a teacher' generates a set of needs, which partly differ from the set generated by the goal 'to live as a farmer in the country'. Liss argues that as different goals generate different sets of needs, a clearly defined goal is therefore a prerequisite for reasonable assessment of need. He sums up the teleological view of need using the formula that 'there is a need when the goal is not realised and there is a need of a certain thing when this is necessary for realising the goal'. He argues that this formula may be used in characterising a need for not only health care but also every other kind of need: a particular thing is needed in so far as it is necessary for eliminating a certain gap or realising a certain goal. This is a useful model in understanding a want and a need. The concept of need is explored further below in terms of health care and services.

Bradshaw's taxonomy of need

In health care, distinctions exist between patient assessed and provider assessed models. It is at this juncture that Bradshaw's (1972) taxonomy of needs reflects the values and perspectives of different groups. The four types of need as identified by Bradshaw are outlined in Box 5.1.

Bradshaw's model provides both a theoretical and a practical level of needs assessment. At a theoretical level, it is useful in drawing attention to the fact that different definitions of need correspond to various groups in society. Thayer (1973) in a study of social welfare provision concluded that the taxonomy of

Box 5.1   Bradshaw's taxonomy of need.

(1)   *Normative needs*, which are defined in relation to an agreed standard, which is determined by an expert or professional. Those individuals or groups who fall short of this standard are identified as being in need of services. This often reflects the value judgements and interests of professional groups.

(2)   *Felt needs*, on the other hand, are identified by individuals themselves and they are reflected in their aspirations and expectations. As this relies on people's own expectations, lack of awareness, knowledge and technical expertise may result in individuals not recognising that they do in fact have a need (Hawtin et al. 1994).

(3)   *Expressed need* is a felt need turned into action. Expressed need is what economists call the demand for a service. People do not demand services unless they feel they need them, but it is common for felt need not to be expressed by demand. Hence, health service planners commonly use demand as a measure of need. For example, waiting lists are often taken as a measure of expressed need or demand. However, Hawtin et al. (1994) argue that as expressed needs reflect current provision and availability, this may not constitute an accurate picture of need per se.

(4)   *Comparative need* refers to the needs of a group of individuals compared to those of another group with similar characteristics. For example, a large number of studies have been carried out to identify characteristics such as low income, unemployment and lone parenthood that are associated with poor health. Comparative need at a population level is the difference between services provided in two different areas, weighted to take account of the factors known to increase the risk of poor health.

needs was a useful way to demarcate different approaches to assessment, but there was little methodological evidence to suggest that the concepts could be operationalised in a meaningful way. Most academic commentators view need as a relative and subjective concept (Bradshaw 1977). It is believed that there is no such thing as objective needs (Harding et al. 1987); rather there are simply different definitions of need held by different groups in society. As this is prone to confusion concerning its objectivity, it can be argued that needs are not only subjective but also relative to a particular time and place.

Doyal and Gough's model of basic and intermediate needs

Doyal and Gough (1991), however, believe that there are objective needs, which are common to everyone – which are universal needs. Their model is based on the notion that the ultimate goal of all human beings is to be able to participate fully in society. In order to do this, they argue that two basic needs must be met: the *need for physical health* and the *need for autonomy*.

Their argument is based on the belief that these two needs are not relative to a particular historical era or to a particular country and they are not subjective value judgements. They maintain that there is a moral imperative to meet fundamental human needs. Hence the two basic needs for health and autonomy are not only the prerequisites for participation in society, but also fundamental rights of all human beings.

Doyal and Gough go further and identify different levels of need. In addition to the two basic needs for health and autonomy, there exist a number of 'intermediate needs', which must be satisfied if the two basic needs are to be protected or improved. They claim that intermediate needs are also universal and objective and list eleven intermediate needs, including adequate food and water, protective housing, non-hazardous work environment, appropriate health care, security in childhood, significant primary relationships, physical security and economic security.

Doyal and Gough argue that basic and intermediate needs can be met in an almost infinite variety of ways. They suggest that evaluation of the range of different policies and services to meet need should take place against the yardstick of how well they meet basic and intermediate needs. In other words, needs assessment is a process of assessing how well people's basic and intermediate needs are being met.

The strength of Doyal and Gough's theoretical approach is that it both provides legitimacy and suggests a particular type of methodological framework for the kinds of auditing or profiling exercises that are carried out by many health professionals (Robinson and Elkan 1996). However, this model does not provide a solution to the fact that different groups in society have different ideas about what their most important needs are, nor does it provide a framework or procedure for assessing and meeting their needs.

Systematic approaches to needs assessment

The term needs assessment has been used to describe a variety of concepts relating to the relationship between service provision and service users (Harding et al. 1987). The concept of need and its assessment is a complex process and the definition of need has many interpretations. Orr (1985) provides an initial interpretation that reveals the multiple meanings attached to the concept, defining need as 'social, relative and evaluative': social in being defined according to standards of communal life, relative in that its meaning will vary between people and societies, and evaluative in that it is based on values and judgements. For many years, people with a learning disability were kept in hospital with the belief that their needs would be better served by secluding them and providing them with a protective environment. Due to changes in social policy, there has been a shift in the service provision for these people, which has led to professionals articulating the need for better health care and better services for these people.

Professionals in the field of learning disability have used the terms needs and needs assessment differently. Needs assessment has been used to explain (1) 'needs for services' as well as (2) 'needs of individual people with learning disability' (Baldwin 1986). In the first category, needs assessment has been employed to describe a method that estimates the usage of existing services by a large number of people with learning disability. In the second category, individual people are given assistance to complete a needs assessment for themselves in order to determine individual services. These two different approaches produce very dissimilar patterns of development. The services that are planned and provided for individuals (rather than for large groups of people) allow more opportunities for localised, flexible and personalised approaches (Baldwin 1986).

Needs assessment has always been a priority issue for those concerned with community health (Billings and Cowley 1995) and a wide range of needs assessment approaches are available. More broadly, sociologists, epidemiologists and health economists have each defined need from their own perspectives. These approaches and their contribution to needs assessment are reviewed briefly in the following sections.

Both the epidemiological and economic approaches have their advantages and disadvantages. Epidemiological data can be useful if collected in a systematic manner, providing a balance for the assessment of needs. Similarly, the economic approach is useful in asserting the necessity for priority setting, which could contribute to the understanding of health needs.

The epidemiological approach

Traditionally, the health needs of a population, community or sections of people are articulated by epidemiological studies. With the epidemiological approach, health is seen as the absence of disease and health need is defined in terms of the presence of disease in a population. According to Stevens and Raftery (1992), needs assessment often relies upon the knowledge of three important factors:

(1)   The local prevalence and incidence of disease, ranged by severity. Prevalence – the number of cases per unit population at a point in time, or over a period – is usually the appropriate measure for chronic disease: and incidence – the number of new cases per unit time – is usually appropriate for measuring acute diseases.
(2)   The efficacies of care and care settings available or potentially available to cope with disease (interventions).
(3)   The cost-effectiveness of such interventions.

Information sources for the epidemiological approach include demographic and social data such as local mortality and morbidity statistics, and statistics concerning levels of deprivation, as well as data concerning the effectiveness and cost-effectiveness of services (Robinson and Elkan 1996). Need is thus defined in terms of lives lost, life years lost, morbidity or loss of social functioning.

According to Stevens and Raftery (1992), in the epidemiological method information on the efficacy of health care and health care settings is scarce. They argue that the development of health care has often been characterised by the adaptation of procedures and dogmas with poor accompanying evidence of their efficacy. In addition to this, the mortality and morbidity statistics are often deficient in relating the burden of health problems to health care services. This may be because changes in mortality and morbidity rates reflect not only changes in health care interventions but also changes in public policy and other environmental and social changes. In this context, mortality data may allow us to monitor whether the population is becoming healthier, but a healthier population is not the result solely of the provision of health care services.

As data concerning the effectiveness of services are often lacking, local purchasers of services rely on measures of supply and demand, such as service utilisation rates or waiting lists. Robinson and Elkan (1996) argue that these are proxy measures for effectiveness. It is based on the assumption that if there is a great demand for services (as measured through waiting lists) or if the service is heavily used (as measured through service utilisation rates) then the services must be effective. Service utilisation records are therefore used as one indicator of need, reflecting the government's view that the public express their need for health care through demand for existing services.

The economic approach

The economic approach limits needs assessment to purely a technical exercise within the current system and ignores the contribution of other services. Health economists point out that the capacity to benefit from health services is always going to be far greater than the resources at our disposal to implement every possible beneficial intervention. Economists stress the need to choose between benefit and outcomes and to identify who is receiving beneficial service and who is not. This is based on the notion that 'no society can afford to offer all its members all the health care that might possibly do them some good. Each society has therefore to establish priorities, that is, it has to decide who will get what and, by implication, who will go without' (Williams 1993, p. 834).

This reflects the QALYs (quality adjusted life years), which focus on the outcomes or consequences of health care interventions based on utilitarian principles. According to Robinson and Elkan (1996), 'QALYs were devised by economists because it was recognised that much of the medical and nursing care is given for conditions which are not life threatening, and that therefore for some conditions, "cure" is neither a realistic nor an appropriate objective' (p. 124). Hence, the need for outcome measures is based on a combination of the quality and quantity of life.

This certainly introduces the question of health rationing in health needs assessment. Robinson and Elkan (1996) point out that if health care resources are to be allocated on the basis of 'need' or on the basis of an 'ability to benefit' from health care, this would lead to determining priorities between competing claims with limited resources. Vulnerable groups such as people with learning disabilities might come into this equation, if limited resources need to be shared between acute medical facilities and long-term care for people with learning disabilities.

Box 5.2   The framework of the MRC Needs for Care Assessment.

The MRC Needs for Care Assessment is designed for people with mental illness who are living in the community. It is based on three conceptual levels (Wing, 1972, 1978, 1986):

(1) The *first* is that of 'social disablement', measured in terms of lowered physical, psychological and social functioning compared with what would ordinarily be expected, in a particular society, of, or for, a particular individual.
(2) The *second* level is concerned with methods of treatment or care that are thought to be effective and acceptable means of helping to reduce or contain the components of social disablement. These include medication, training, other treatment programmes and various kinds of support and shelter.
(3) The *third* conceptual level involves the services needed to provide treatment or care for people who are socially disabled. In this context, services refer to the organisational structures that facilitate the identification of people in need and the delivery of appropriate treatment or care for people who are socially disabled (Brewin et al. 1987).

A model for needs assessment

The conceptual model of needs assessment discussed in this chapter is based on the studies of Marshall (1994) and Marshall et al. (1995) which discuss the methodology for a systematic process of measuring need. Marshall's model of needs assessment, the *Cardinal Needs Schedule*, is an adapted version of the Medical Research Council (MRC) Needs for Care Assessment (Brewin et al. 1987) model of needs assessment used in adult psychiatry (Box 5.2).

In the MRC Needs for Care Assessment, Brewin and colleagues argue that needs for health and medical care cannot be properly assessed and compared between settings without an explicit model of care that states the assumptions behind the development of the instrument. Such an explicit model permits both the ideology of an instrument and the logic of individual judgements to be freely inspected. Brewin et al.'s vision is based on the belief that one cannot realistically measure the needs of specific groups without clear views about therapeutic and rehabilitative processes.

The MRC Needs for Care Assessment provides an outline model of ideal clinical practice in the care of the long-term mentally ill. According to Brewin et al. (1987), this model has three elements.

(1) The patient's clinical and social functioning should be regularly and systematically assessed in order to identify areas of improvement or deterioration. General goals consist of amelioration of symptoms and distress, and improvement in social and occupational skills.
(2) An identified deficit or problem should prompt a list of potential interventions, ranging from active therapy or training to the provision of support and shelter. The failure or only partial success of one intervention should lead automatically, after a specified period, to trials of other interventions from the list.

(3) Failure or only partial success of all appropriate forms of care should trigger future intervention at regular intervals in the hope that the patient would be more able to utilise help or that the help offered would be more in accord with the patient's own priorities. Magi and Allander (1981) suggest that need statements may describe an actual state of affairs, but they also depend on implicit or explicit value systems that determine which states of affairs are considered acceptable and which course of action should be considered. This supports the notion that needs can never be objectively defined, but must be understood in terms of the person or group making the judgement (Brewin et al. 1987).

Based on this model, the MRC Needs for Care Assessment puts forward its definition of need for care as follows:

(1) A need is present when (a) a patient's functioning falls below some minimum specified level, and (b) this is due to some remediable or potentially remediable cause.
(2) A need as defined in (a) is met when it has attracted some or at least partly effective intervention, and when no interventions of greater potential effectiveness exist.
(3) A need as defined in (a) is unmet when it has attracted only partly effective or no intervention and when other interventions of greater potential effectiveness exist.

The MRC Needs for Care Assessment: structures and processes

As identified previously, the MRC needs assessment procedure follows from the initial identification of a significant problem in clinical or social functioning. The MRC schedule measures need in three steps:

(1) An area of functioning is selected.
(2) Whether the patient has a problem is assessed.
(3) Whether the problem identified is a need is then determined.

The first step is the assessment of functioning, which involves assessing the individual's symptoms and behaviour problems, and their personal and social skills. An area of functioning is an aspect of life in which patients with a chronic illness or disability commonly have problems. Table 5.1 shows the areas of functioning classified as symptoms, behaviour problems, skills and abilities. Each area of functioning is associated with a list of 'items of care' (such as remedial training or medication) which experts in psychiatric rehabilitation believe are suitable interventions for a problem in the area.

The second step determines whether a problem is present in an area of functioning, and for this, behavioural and psychiatric rating scales are used. These scales include standardised ways of describing a patient's mental state

Table 5.1   Areas of functioning and intervention considered by the LDCNS.

No.	Area of functioning	Interventions	No.	Area of functioning	Interventions
1	Psychotic symptoms	Psychiatric assessment Physical investigations Medication Monitoring of medication Domestic visits Support and reassurance Behavioural family therapy Nursing care plan	5	Epilepsy	Medical assessment Medication Nursing care plan
2	Anxiety/depressive symptoms	Psychiatric assessment Medication Nursing care plan Psychological treatment Support	6	Medical problems	Specialist assessment Specific treatment Coping advice (carer) Coping advice (patient) Nursing care plan Advice on aids
3	Dangerous or destructive behaviour	Psychiatric assessment Supervision Nursing care plan Medication Behavioural intervention Environmental manipulation Anger management	7	Sensory impairment	Specialist assessment Sensory aids
			8	Drug and alcohol abuse	Specialist assessment Support and counselling Self-help group Detoxification at home Admission for detoxification Advice on safe practices Behavioural intervention Medication
4	Self-harm	Psychiatric assessment Supervision Nursing care plan Medication Behavioural intervention Environmental manipulation	9	Sleep problems	Advice Nursing care plan Medication
			10	Eating problems	Advice on healthy eating Nursing care plan Behavioural intervention Dietician assessment

11	Socially embarrassing behaviour	Advice Nursing care plan Behavioural intervention Supervision and monitoring Incontinence aids Medication
12	Side effects of medication	Psychiatric assessment Reduction or change in medication Medication Monitoring of side effects
13	Communication skills and language	Assessment of speech or language Literacy training Sign language training Speech therapy Special aids
14	Domestic skills	Home help Remedial training Specialist assessment Special domestic aids
15	Hygiene and dressing	Remedial training Supervised bathing and dressing
16	Mobility and use of amenities	Remedial training Special transport Specialist assessment Special aids
17	Social life	Coping advice Structured day activity Sheltered leisure Community social activity Activity support worker Social skills training
18	Employment	Job coaching Employment training Paid work Sheltered or voluntary work
19	Money management	External control of finance Remedial training Welfare advice or representation
20	Safety	Advice Nursing care plan Supervision and monitoring Behavioural intervention Environmental manipulation
21	Dementia	Psychiatric assessment Nursing care plan Supervision and monitoring
22	Accommodation	Own flat or house Unstaffed group home Staffed group home Family placement

using the Present State Examination (PSE) (Wing et al. 1974), the Social Behaviour Schedule (Wykes and Sturt 1986) and the Abnormal Involuntary Movement Scale (NIMH 1976). When a patient's score on the appropriate rating scale for an area of functioning is greater than a predetermined threshold, a 'problem' is said to be present in that area.

The third step determines the 'need status' for those areas of functioning in which a problem is identified by standardised ratings. A 'need' in the MRC Schedule is defined as a problem for which an intervention has not been given an adequate, recent trial. The need status of an area thus depends on whether all suitable interventions on the list of interventions for that area have been offered. Thus according to the MRC Schedule, an 'unmet need' exists when there is at least one such intervention on the list. A 'met need' exists either when a partially effective intervention is being offered and no other suitable intervention is available, or when a problem has recently been resolved following the provision of an intervention. A 'no need' (as defined by the MRC Schedule) exists when all suitable interventions have been given a reasonable trial, but have not been effective. Thus each person assessed by the MRC schedule will have a rating of x unmet needs, y met needs and z no needs, where $x + y + z = 20$, there being 20 areas of functioning (Marshall 1994).

The Camberwell Assessment of Need (CAN)

The MRC Needs for Care Assessment provided a major lead for the development of further needs assessment schedules in mental health care. One such schedule, the Camberwell Assessment of Need (CAN) developed by Phelan et al. (1995), claims to fulfil the statutory obligation of services to conduct comprehensive needs assessment, which can assist the routine care and treatment of people with severe mental illness. The CAN model has been adapted to people with learning disabilities, and is known as the Camberwell Assessment of Needs for adults with Developmental and Intellectual Disability (CANDID) (Xenitidis et al. 2000). This model of encouraging systematic and regular needs assessment to shape care plans has many similarities to the MRC Needs for Care Assessment and hence this requires some discussion in this context. The principle of needs assessment used by CAN and CANDID is based on the following ideas:

(1) Everyone has needs and although people with mental illness have some specific needs, most of their needs are similar to those of people not suffering from mental illness. The CAN reflects this notion by incorporating a wide range of human needs, such as shelter and the company of other people, as well as those specific to people suffering from mental illness.

(2) People with mental illness may have multiple needs, which are not recognised by mental health services. Hence, Phelan et al. state that a priority of CAN is to identify, rather than describe in depth, serious needs, since

more detailed and specialist assessments can be conducted in specific areas when required.

(3) Needs assessment should be both an integral part of routine clinical practice and a component of service evaluation, so the instrument could be easily learned and practised by a wide range of clinical staff.

(4) Staff on their own should not define needs.

The CAN and CANDID use 22 areas of functioning: food, accommodation, housing skills, self-care, occupation, physical health, psychotic symptoms, information about condition and treatment, psychological distress, safety to self, safety to others, alcohol, drugs, company of others, intimate relationships, sexual expression, child care, basic education, telephone, transport, money and finally welfare benefits. The CAN follows an identical structure for all the areas and each area of need includes four sections. The first section establishes whether there is a need, by asking about difficulties in that area. Responses are rated on a three-point scale: 0 – no serious problem; 1 – no serious problems or moderate problem because of continuing intervention (met need); 2 – current serious problem (unmet need). The second section asks about help received from friends, relatives and other informal carers. The third section asks about how much help the person is getting, and how much help he or she needs from local statutory services. All ratings of help are on a four-point scale: 0 – none; 1 – low; 2 – moderate; 3 – high. Phelan et al. claim that CAN is a comprehensive and relatively brief needs assessment tool, which is easy for a wide range of staff to learn to use.

Limitations of the MRC Needs Schedule

The MRC Needs for Care Assessment is an important innovation in the assessment of mental health and personal care needs (Marshall et al. 1995), but some researchers have identified certain practical limitations. Holloway (1991) found it necessary to make changes to the procedures recommended by Brewin and colleagues, while some other researchers familiar with the schedule proposed the development of modified approaches (Pryce et al. 1993) or new approaches (Thornicroft et al. 1993). The MRC Schedule is time consuming (Hogg and Marshall 1992) because of the number of standardised instruments and owing to the administration and decision-making process (Marshall 1994). It recommends that the views of patients and carers should be taken into account when making ratings of need, but the authors fail to provide adequate guidelines for this purpose.

This theme was further explored by Hogg and Marshall (1992) and Marshall et al. (1995), who suggested three main reasons why a needs schedule should explicitly and systematically elicit the views of patients and their carers:

(1) The views of patients and carers are elicited and taken into account in everyday clinical practice; hence a schedule that aims to emulate clinical practice should likewise elicit and consider these views.

(2) If a needs assessment is to be standardised, there should be explicit guidance on how the views of patients and carers are to be elicited and how these views should be taken into account when rating need. Marshall et al. (1995) suggest that this would enable other researchers to consider the rules for incorporating the views of patients and carers into the ratings.

(3) It has been found that patients often regard 'problems' identified by clinicians as unimportant, particularly in relation to life skills (MacCarthy et al. 1986). Hence, it is important to establish explicitly the patient's willingness to co-operate in this process.

Structure of the Learning Disability version of the Cardinal Needs Schedule (LDCNS)

The development of the LDCNS is based on the systematic assessment of needs using the Cardinal Needs Schedule (CNS) (Marshall 1994; Marshall et al. 1995), which provides a four-stage model of needs assessment (Fig. 5.1). This consists of:

(1) Assessment of functioning of the individual's symptoms, behaviour problems, personal and social skills in a number of areas of functioning, in which one might be prepared to intervene in principle.

(2) Determining whether problems exist in any of these areas of functioning.

(3) Applying a set of criteria to determine whether it is appropriate to act on an identified problem.

(4) Determining the need for appropriate intervention in the areas of functioning, where problems are identified.

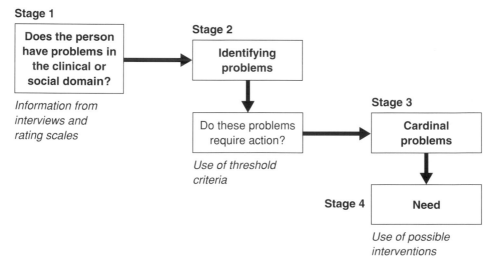

Fig. 5.1 A working model for the Learning Disability version of the Cardinal Needs Schedule (LDCNS).

Stage 1: Identification of areas of functioning and problems

Areas of functioning are aspects of life in which chronic patients commonly have problems (Marshall 1994). These fall into two groups: (1) the *clinical domain*, covering symptoms and behaviour problems, for example psychotic symptoms, physical illness and side effects of medication; and (2) the *social domain*, covering skills and abilities, for example education, social life and domestic skills.

For the LDCNS, twenty-two areas of functioning exist, twelve in the clinical domain and ten in the social domain (see Table 5.1). Lists of appropriate interventions were also developed for each area of functioning in consultation with clinicians working with people with learning disabilities.

Stage 2: Assessment of problems

The assessment process of the CNS should be relatively simple and short, be acceptable to the service users and providers and standardised (Marshall 1994; Marshall et al. 1995). Such a process should permit straightforward ratings of problems in each area of functioning which could then be compared with criteria provided by the schedule.

Standardised instruments are used to measure the client's performance in areas of psychological, psychiatric and social functioning. Ratings of performance in each area of functioning are then compared with criteria set by the schedule. *If an individual's performance in an area falls below the standard set by these criteria, then a problem is said to be present.* For the data collection process on behaviour and mental state, the Manchester Scale and the Rehabilitation Evaluation Hall and Baker (REHAB) were used. These two standardised instruments were chosen because they were simple to use and already their use in the CNS has proven their effectiveness in measuring the behaviour and mental state of clients.

The Psychiatric Assessment Schedule for Adults with a Developmental Disability (PAS-ADD) (Moss et al. 1993) was used for psychiatric interview. Moss et al. (1993) suggest that an experienced interviewer would be able to complete the PAS-ADD interviews in 30 minutes. PAS-ADD covers a wide spectrum of mental health items designed to detect these symptoms in people with dual diagnosis. However, there are some limitations. For example, PAS-ADD does not have a section on expansive mood to detect hypomania (Moss et al. 1996) nor does it provide a severity score at the end of the interview covering all the items in the schedule. The data from PAS-ADD interviews were used to rate the Revised Manchester Scale (Krawiecka et al. 1977). The rationale for using the Manchester Scale in this study is based on (1) its quick and easy styles of interpreting the scores and (2) its ability to provide severity scores for symptoms.

In order to assess the skills and behaviours of clients, REHAB (Baker and Hall 1988), a standardised behaviour scale for rating living skills and behaviour, was used. REHAB was used in the learning disability version of the

CNS because it is quick and easy to use by carers and in community settings for people with chronic mental illness (Hewitt 1983).

The other standardised interviews developed for the needs assessment schedule include the client opinion interview and the carer stress interview. The client opinion interview is a semi-structured interview schedule designed to identify problems in the areas of functioning. The carer stress interview is a semi-structured interview schedule to rate the carer's stress in relation to the client's anxiety or depression, self-harm or aggression, health status, challenging behaviour, domestic skills, finance and welfare, social life, transport and amenities, and hygiene and dressing.

Three additional instruments for collecting data from carers and the case notes of clients were developed for the LDCNS:

(1) The *additional information questionnaire*: this was devised specifically for the CNS (Marshall et al. 1995). It consists of items concerned with medical, psychiatric and social history (for example, it records whether the person is in employment or if he/she has been arrested in the past year for socially embarrassing behaviour). This questionnaire is completed after consulting the person's notes and the main carer.

(2) *Supplementary questions*: this questionnaire is designed specifically for people with learning disability to identify any problems in areas such as dementia, socially embarrassing behaviour, domestic skills, mobility and use of amenities and safety. Carers are asked information relating to these questions.

(3) The *auxiliary schedule*: this is specifically designed to record the results of the various tests given during the interview process. These consist of tests for vision and hearing, alcohol and drug screening, and the patient's height and weight for calculating the body mass index (BMI).

Stage 3: Identifying cardinal problems

The LDCNS uses a battery of instruments to identify the problems of clients and carers and a range of standardised interview schedules and rating scales to assess the behaviour and mental state of the clients. As well as the additional information questionnaire, supplementary questions and the auxiliary schedule, these include the following:

(1) *The client opinion interview*: this is a semistructured interview schedule used to seek the opinion of the client and to identify problems in the areas of functioning.

(2) *The carer stress interview*: this is a semistructured interview schedule used to determine the stress factors for the carer in caring for the client, to rate the carer's stress in relation to the client's anxiety or depression, self-harm or aggression, health status, challenging behaviour, domestic skills, finance and welfare, social life, transport and amenities, and hygiene and dressing.

(3) *The Manchester Scale* (Krawiecka et al. 1977): this is used to measure the mental state of the patient and side effects of medication. This is a five-point rating scale, designed to measure the severity of psychiatric symptoms in chronic patients. The scale covers depression, anxiety, coherently expressed delusions, hallucinations, incoherence and irrelevance of speech, poverty of speech, blunted affect and psychomotor retardation. In addition to this, it has a section for rating drug side effects. The five-point scale used for rating the mental state of the patient consists of the following: 0 (symptoms absent), 1 (mild symptoms present), 2 (moderate symptoms present), 3 (marked symptoms present) and 4 (severe symptoms present).

(4) *Rehabilitation Evaluation Hall and Baker (REHAB)* (Baker and Hall 1988): this is a standardised behaviour scale which rates living skills, such as communication and self-care (general behaviour), and the frequency of disruptive behaviours such as violence, self-harm and shouting (deviant behaviour).

(5) *The Psychiatric Assessment Schedule for Adults with a Developmental Disability (PAS-ADD)* (Moss et al. 1993): this is a psychiatric interview schedule standardised for people with learning disabilities.

The CNS was required to determine whether the problems identified were cardinal problems, *which are problems requiring an action*. In clinical settings, not all problems may require an action, and hence it is important to identify the problems that do require action using appropriate criteria. This involved establishing a set of criteria as to whether it was appropriate to act on an identified problem (see Box 5.3).

Box 5.3 Criteria for identifying cardinal problems.

The client opinion interview determines:

(1) the client's attitude towards receiving help in a number of problem areas;
(2) whether the client wishes to change his/her accommodation; and
(3) whether the client is distressed by any current physical problems.

The carer stress interview determines whether the carer finds that the client's behaviour:

(1) is causing considerable worry or anxiety;
(2) is significantly upsetting; or
(3) is disruptive because of the amount of time spent dealing with it.

In order to decide if it is appropriate to act on the cardinal problem, the schedule provides three criteria:

(1) the co-operation criterion (Is the client willing to accept help for the problem?);
(2) the carer stress criterion (Do people caring for the client express severe anxiety or annoyance as a result of the problem?); and
(3) the severity criterion (Is the nature and severity of the problem such that the client's health and safety or the safety of others are at risk?).

Table 5.2   Criteria used for rating cardinal problems.

Area of functioning	Criteria		
	Severity	Co-operation	Carer stress
Clinical domain			
Psychotic symptoms	Yes	No	No
Dementia	Yes	No	No
Anxiety or depression	Yes	No	Yes
Dangerous or destructive behaviour	Yes	No	Yes
Self-harm	Yes	No	Yes
Epilepsy	Yes	No	No
Physical illness	Yes	Yes	Yes
Sensory impairment	No	Yes	No
Drug and alcohol abuse	No	Yes	No
Sleep problems	No	Yes	Yes
Socially embarrassing behaviour	No	Yes	Yes
Side effects of medication	Yes	No	Yes
Social domain			
Eating problems	No	Yes	Yes
Communication skills and language	Yes	Yes	No
Domestic skills	No	Yes	Yes
Hygiene and dressing	No	No	Yes
Mobility and use of amenities	Yes	Yes	No
Social life	No	Yes	Yes
Employment	No	Yes	No
Money management	No	Yes	Yes
Safety	Yes	No	No
Accommodation	N/A	N/A	N/A

Marshall suggests that the three criteria identified in Box 5.3 are not invariably applied in each area of functioning (see Table 5.2). The co-operation criterion is applied in areas where a person is likely to be offered some form of skill training as an intervention (for example an occupation). The carer stress criterion is applied in areas where the problem could cause stress to carers and where there are steps that could reasonably be taken to relieve this stress, whether or not the patient is able to give his/her consent (for example socially embarrassing behaviour). The severity criterion is applied in areas where a problem could present a risk to the health or safety of the patient, or the safety of others (for example dangerous or destructive behaviour); in such cases interventions can be offered whether the person consents or not.

Stage 4: Identifying cardinal needs

For each kind of cardinal problem there is a list of suitable interventions, which are predetermined and objectively defined. A cardinal problem is identified as *a need when there are one or more suitable interventions that have not been offered in the past year* (see Table 5.1 for possible interventions).

In the needs assessment process, the clinician is required to allocate each potential intervention to one of four possible categories:

(1) The category 'offered' is applied when an intervention has been offered in the past year.
(2) The category 'not offered' is applied when an intervention is deemed appropriate, but has not been offered in the past year.
(3) The category 'inappropriate' is applied when there is a strong clinical reason for withholding the intervention from a particular client.
(4) The category 'suspended' is applied when an intervention has been offered so recently that its effect cannot be evaluated.

When there are one or more interventions that have not been offered, then a need is said to be present. In many cases, clinicians may have offered all the possible interventions and the need may still be present. The LDCNS identifies this scenario, which is crucial in clinical practice, which states that 'if all possible interventions have been offered and the cardinal problem is present, then the cardinal problem persists despite intervention (PDI)' (Marshall et al. 1995).

The CNS uses a computer program called Autoneed, which runs with Microsoft Windows 95. Autoneed is a stand-alone program, where data are stored in an industry database format (Microsoft Access). The Autoneed program is used in four steps:

(1) Data from the standardised instruments are entered into the database by investigators or secretarial staff.
(2) Autoneed automatically identifies objective problems and cardinal problems (corresponding to stages 1 and 2 of the LDCNS), and goes on to provide the investigator with tables of suitable interventions for each cardinal problem that has been identified.
(3) The investigator rates these interventions and Autoneed decides whether a need is present (corresponding to stage 3).
(4) The data on need (corresponding to stage 4) are automatically stored in a table of results, so that an immediate analysis can be performed using preprogrammed routines.

The needs assessment process

The methods of needs assessment used in practice mainly consist of the use of checklists for observing skills and behaviours of clients. The needs assessment process adopted by the LDCNS and CANDID attempt to provide a detailed picture of the number of needs and the suitable interventions that could be implemented to meet these needs. The structure of needs assessment used by CANDID is similar to the LDCNS in the initial stages, but important differences lie in the use of standardised instruments, computer software, criteria and thresholds used to determine whether problems identified require interventions and provision of a protocol of interventions.

The stages of the LDCNS, that is identifying problems, identifying cardinal problems and identifying need, provide a structured and systematic method of assessing the needs of people with dual diagnosis through the use of standardised interview schedules and rating scales. The 22 areas of functioning chosen for LDCNS provide a template for identifying the problems and thus allowing the assessor to focus on these specific areas for his or her client group. For example, the assessor will be able to focus on anxiety and identify the objective problems in this area of functioning. The use of standardised interview schedules and rating scales such as PAS-ADD, the Manchester Scale and the REHAB to identify the objective problems allows a format for systematically gathering information through the incorporation of contemporary measures in the field of learning disability and mental health.

The second stage, that of identifying cardinal problems, offers a model for classifying problems that require action. Indeed, not all the problems of clients require action in everyday clinical practice. Hence, this stage is important in deciding what are the main problems identified that require action, thus making best use of clinical and other resources available (Marshall 1994). In working with people with learning disabilities, paid and family carers are required to 'act in the best interests' of the person and therefore it is especially important to acknowledge the conflicts of interest. The use of a systematic account of the views of clients and carers for deciding cardinal problems does indeed help to address this problem (see Box 5.4).

The use of these criteria places the service user and his or her carers at the centre of identifying those problems in the clinical and social domain with which they may require help. Therefore, clients and their carers are involved in the decision-making process concerning their cardinal problems and a

Box 5.4 Example of the needs assessment process using the LDCNS.

Using the LDCNS, person B was rated as having a need for intervention owing to anxiety and/or depression. This was derived as follows:

- *Stage 1 (identifying problems)*
  On the Manchester Scale, person B had a score of 2, indicating anxiety and/or depression.
- *Stage 2 (problems requiring action)*
  At this stage, the problems were rated as cardinal problems on the grounds of the Manchester Scale showing a score of 2 for neurotic symptoms, indicating the severity criterion, and a carer stress score of 1, indicating that the carer is experiencing stress or annoyance as a result of person B's anxiety.
- *Stage 3 (choosing intervention)*
  At this stage, the list of suitable interventions for this area was reviewed. Interventions such as psychiatric assessment and medication and support were offered, but psychological intervention was not offered. Hence the person was rated as having a need for psychological intervention for anxiety disorder.

standardised process of needs assessment is also maintained. Slade (1994) argues that with needs assessment being an integral part of social and medical care, assessment techniques must take account of both user and staff views. This is an important step because it reduces the professional bias, which might otherwise contribute to the process of needs assessment.

There can also be situations in clinical practice where a need continues to exist for some client(s) regardless of the interventions offered. For example, in the area of anxiety and/or depression, for person G, a need for intervention was persisting despite offering all the appropriate interventions suggested in the schedule (psychiatric assessment, medication, nursing care plan, psychological intervention and support). The identification of a problem persisting despite intervention (PDI) is indeed a significant step in the process of needs assessment because this could lead to further examination of or evaluation of the possible reasons for the existence of various needs despite intervention for treatment. This provides a clear focus for evaluating the outcomes of the interventions offered.

Needs do not exist in the real world in a ready-made and already labelled style; hence, to describe needs we require some standards or criteria (Charles and Webb 1986). Thus, the assessment of needs of people with dual diagnosis using the LDCNS employs a set of criteria that can be further verified, adapted or improved. The output of the LDCNS is easy to interpret because needs and PDI offer two simple ways of appraising the performance of a particular service. Marshall et al. (1995) argue that the ratings of 'need' are a measure of intervention delivery indicating how far a service has not been delivering suitable interventions. The ratings of PDI, on the other hand, are a measure of 'intervention failure', thus showing how far the interventions have proven ineffective.

From the reliability study of the LDCNS (Raghavan et al. 2004), it is possible to identify the key clinical and social needs of people with dual diagnosis. These consist of:

- Assessment and diagnosis
- Behaviour and psychological and pharmacological interventions
- Skill teaching for life and living
- Health screening, access to health services and nursing care
- Housing and supported accommodation facilities
- Promoting self-esteem through work, leisure and social life
- Help with communication
- Support and training for family and paid carers.

The implementation of care management puts the onus of service provision on the assessment of individual needs of service users and carers. In this context, the question often asked is how nurses should go about assessing and meeting the needs of people with dual diagnosis. The policy guidelines stress the need for interagency working in the care and service provision of people with dual diagnosis. Evaluations of care management suggest that 'both health commissioners and local authority commissioners must have a role in setting the strategic framework within which care management will operate. Many localities lack a coherent service strategy for learning disability and challenging behaviour' (Greig et al. 1996, p. 9). In such a climate, it remains to be seen how joint assessment between health and social services will be implemented locally and at an individual level. Hence, the processes of joint working through the operationalisation of a systematic and structured approach of needs assessment for people with dual diagnosis should form a key part of the nursing role. The needs assessment process of the LDCNS and CANDID provides a conceptual model for systematically assessing the complex individual needs of this population and in order to plan interventions.

Clinicians including nurses and key service providers eloquently articulate the underfunding of services for people with learning disabilities. Commissioners of health and social services often argue that resources are limited and that they have to work within a tight budget. The ideological concept of providing a package of services based on individual needs through person-centred planning does not tally with the reality of finite resources struggling to cope with the overwhelming needs of people with learning disabilities in general, let alone people with dual diagnosis. This leads to the question of whether all the identified needs can be met within the overstretched financial resources of the service providers. The process of needs assessment of people with learning difficulties and their carers might provide an undue expectation that services might be able to meet their needs, which may be far from the reality in many localities.

From a pragmatic perspective, service providers are not equipped to meet all the assessed needs due to the shortage of resources, but there is a strong case for targeting resources at high quality interventions which effect significant changes in service quality and appropriateness (Cambridge 1999). This, if used effectively, can help with the targeting of needs and effective utilisation of resources, thereby reducing the burden of the number of extra contractual referrals (ECR). Consequently, this should mobilise the creation of high quality developers of needs-led services to address the complex needs of people with dual diagnosis.

Another issue relating to the needs of people with dual diagnosis is that of accurate case detection and assessment. A number of factors influence the detection and diagnostic process. As mental health disorders do not have clear-cut definitions, diagnosis will depend on the interaction of a variety of factors such as what people say they are experiencing, what others say about them, how they are seen to behave and the history of their complaint (Moss 1999). As detection and diagnosis heavily rely on third party reports due to the communication barriers of a significant majority of people with learning disabilities, it is important to utilise a structured framework to enhance this process. Nursing assessments using screening tools for mental health disorder, clinical interviews with carers, clients and their relatives and extensive data collection on behavioural and social aspects of the person's life will help with detection and diagnosis. This will contribute to a comprehensive method of data collection relating to decline in the level of functioning due to the impact of a specific mental health disorder.

The overlap of challenging behaviour with mental health disorder adds further confusion to the debate regarding diagnosis and detection. The behavioural overlap with symptoms of mental health disorders in people with learning disabilities poses more questions than answers. For instance, how can we detect the aggravation of behaviour problems as a result of mental health disorders? As the challenging behaviour manifests over a longer term in this population, how can we differentiate between a mental health symptom and a learned inappropriate behaviour? The separation of the psychological aspects affecting the personality of an individual with learning disabilities and the mental health symptoms is a real challenge for psychiatrists, nurses and other clinicians working in this field. Hence, it is important to collect information relating to a range of life situations using standardised procedures, thereby narrowing the factors and behaviours that require in-depth investigation.

In order to provide better services for people with dual diagnosis, clinicians should concentrate on identifying the need for assessment and intervention. This should help service providers to focus on specific needs and symptoms and to monitor the outcome of interventions and behaviour change over a period of time. Simpson (1997) suggests that a systematic approach to the development of services for people with dual diagnosis should proceed with an assessment of need. Hence, the identification of need is a prerequisite for service planning and delivery.

Conclusion

In this chapter we have explored the concept of need and its assessment. The concept of need and its interpretations helps to enlighten the subjective nature of need and its assessment in health and social care. The thrust of the community care legislation is the identification of needs through appropriate assessments and planning individualised services based on needs assessment. We have highlighted the process and mechanism of a systematic approach to assess the clinical and social needs of people with learning disabilities and mental health disorder.

References

Baker, R. and Hall, J. (1988) *Users Manual: Rehabilitation Evaluation Hall and Baker (REHAB)*. Aberdeen: Vine Publishing.

Baldwin, S. (1986) Problem with needs – where theory meets practice. *Disability, Handicap and Society*, **1**, 139–145.

Billings, R. and Cowley, S. (1995) Approaches to community needs assessment: a literature review. *Journal of Advanced Nursing*, **22**, 721–730.

Bradshaw, J. (1972) The concept of social need. *New Society*, 30 March, 640–643.

Bradshaw, J. (1977) The concept of social need. In: N. Gilbert and H. Specht (Eds) *Planning for Social Welfare Issues: Models and Tasks*. New Jersey: Prentice Hall.

Brewin, C.R., Wing, J.K., Mangen, S.P., Brugha, T.S. and MacCarthy, B. (1987) Principles and practice of measuring needs in the long-term mentally ill: the MRC Needs for Care Assessment. *Psychological Medicine*, **17**, 971–981.

Cambridge, P. (1999) The state of care management in services for people with mental retardation in the UK. In: N. Bouras (Ed.) *Psychiatric and Behavioural Disorders in Developmental Disabilities and Mental Retardation*. Cambridge: Cambridge University Press.

Campbell, T.D. (1974) Humanity before justice. *British Journal of Political Science*, **4**, 1–16.

Charles, S.T. and Webb, A.L. (1986) *The Economic Approach to Social Policy*. Brighton: Wheatsheaf Books.

Department of Health (1989) *Caring for People: Community Care in the Next Decade and Beyond*. Cmnd 849. London: HMSO.

Department of Health (1990) *The National Health Service and Community Care Act*. London: HMSO.

Department of Health (1991a) *Assessment Systems and Community Care*. London: HMSO.

Department of Health (1991b) *Care Management and Assessment: Practitioner's Guide*. London: HMSO.

Department of Health (1994) *Review of Health and Social Services for Mentally Disordered Offenders and Others Requiring Similar Services: People with Learning Disabilities (Mental Handicap) or with Autism* (Chairman: Dr John Reed) Vol. 7. London: HMSO.

Department of Health (2001) *Valuing People: A New Strategy for Learning Disability for the 21st Century*. London: The Stationery Office.

Department of Health and Social Security (1971) *Better Services for the Mentally Handicapped*. Cmnd 4683. London: HMSO.

Doyal, L. and Gough, I. (1991) *A Theory of Human Need*. London: Macmillan.

Greig, R., Cambridge, P. and Rucker, L. (1996) Care management and joint commissioning. In: J. Harris (Ed.) *Purchasing Services for People with Learning Disabilities, Challenging Behaviour and Mental Health Needs*. Kidderminster: British Institute of Learning Disabilities.

Harding, K., Baldwin, S. and Baser, C. (1987) Towards multi-level needs assessment. *Behavioural Psychotherapy*, **15**, 134–143.

Hawtin, M., Hughes, G. and Percy-Smith, J. (1994) *Community Profiling: Auditing Social Needs*. Buckingham: Open University Press.

Hewitt, K.E. (1983) The behaviour of schizophrenic day-patients at home: an assessment by relatives. *Psychological Medicine*, **13**, 885–889.

Hogg, I.L. and Marshall, M. (1992) Can we measure need in the homeless mentally ill? Using the MRC Needs for Care Assessment in hostels for the homeless. *Psychological Medicine*, **22**, 1027–1034.

Holloway, F. (1991) Day care in an inner city II: quality of the services. *British Journal of Psychiatry*, **158**, 810–816.

Krawiecka, M., Goldberg, D. and Vaughan, M. (1977) A standardised psychiatric assessment scale for rating chronic psychiatric patients. *Acta Psychiatrica Scandinavica*, **55**, 299–308.

Liss, P. (1998) Assessing health care need: the conceptual foundation. In: S. Baldwin (Ed.) *Needs Assessment and Community Care: Clinical Practice and Policymaking*. Oxford: Butterworth-Heinemann.

MacCarthy, B., Benson, J. and Brewin, C.R. (1986) Task motivation and problems appraisal in long-term psychiatric patients. *Psychological Medicine*, **16**, 431–438.

Magi, M. and Allander, E. (1981) Towards a theory of perceived and medically defined need. *Sociology of Health and Illness*, **3**, 49–71.

Marshall, M. (1994) How should we measure need? Concept and practice in the development of a standardised assessment schedule. *Philosophy, Psychiatry, and Psychology*, **1**, 27–36.

Marshall, M., Hogg, L.I., Gath, D.H. and Lockwood, A. (1995) The Cardinal Needs Schedule – a modified version of the MRC Needs for Care Assessment Schedule. *Psychological Medicine*, **25**, 605–617.

Maslow, A.H. (1954) *Motivation and Personality*. New York: Harper.

Maslow, A.H. (1970) *Motivation and Personality*, 2nd edn. New York: Harper and Row.

Moss, S. (1999) Assessment of mental health problems. *Tizard Learning Disability Review*, **4**, 14–19.

Moss, S., Patel, P., Prosser, H., et al. (1993) Psychiatric morbidity in older people with moderate and severe learning disability. I: Development and reliability of the patient interview (PAS-ADD). *British Journal of Psychiatry*, **163**, 471–480.

Moss, S., Prosser, H. and Goldberg, D. (1996) Validity of the schizophrenia diagnosis of the Psychiatric Assessment Schedule for Adults with Developmental Disability (PAS-ADD). *British Journal of Psychiatry*, **168**, 359–367.

Murray, A.H. (1938) *Explorations in Personality*. New York: Oxford University Press.

National Institute of Mental Health (NIMH) (1976) *Abnormal Involuntary Movement Scale, ECDEAU Assessment Manual*. Rockville: US Department of Health, Education and Welfare.

Orr, J. (1985) Health visiting and the community. In: K. Luker and J. Orr (Eds) *Health Visiting*. Oxford: Blackwell Scientific.

Phelan, M., Slade, M., Thornicroft, G., et al. (1995) The Camberwell Assessment of Need: the validity and reliability of an instrument to assess the needs of people with severe mental illness. *British Journal of Psychiatry*, **167**, 589–595.

Pryce, I.G., Griffiths, R.D., Gentry, R.M., et al. (1993) How important is the assessment of social skills in current long-stay in-patients? An evaluation of clinical response to needs for assessment, treatment and care in a long-stay psychiatric in-patient population. *British Journal of Psychiatry*, **162**, 498–503.

Raghavan, R., Marshall, M., Lockwood, L. and Duggan, L. (2004) Assessing the needs of people with learning disabilities and mental illness: development of the learning disability version of the Cardinal Needs Schedule. *Journal of Intellectual Disability Research*, **48**, 25–37.

Richards, S. (1994) Making sense of needs assessment. *Research, Policy and Planning*, **12**, 5–8.

Robinson, J. and Elkan, R. (1996) *Health Needs Assessment: Theory and Practice*. London: Churchill Livingston.

Sim, A.J., Love, J. and Lishman, J. (1998) Definitions of need: can disabled people and care professionals agree? *Disability and Society*, **13**, 53–74.

Simpson, N. (1997) Developing mental health services for people with learning disabilities in England. *Tizard Learning Disability Review*, **2**, 35–42.

Slade, M. (1994) Needs assessment. *British Journal of Psychiatry*, **165**, 293–296.

Stevens, A., and Gabbay, J. (1991) Needs assessment. *Health Trends*, **23**, 20–23.

Stevens, A. and Raftery, J. (1992) The purchasers' information requirements on mental health needs and contracting for mental health services. In: G. Thornicroft, C.R. Brewin and J. Wing (Eds) *Measuring Mental Health Needs*. London: Gaskell.

Thayer, R. (1973) Measuring needs in the social services. *Social and Economic Administration*, 7 May, 91–105.

Thornicroft, G., Ward, P. and James, S. (1993) Care management and mental health. *British Medical Journal*, **306**, 768–771.

Wiggins, D. (1987) *Needs, Values and Truth*. Oxford: Basil Blackwell.

Williams, A. (1993) Economics, society and health care ethics. In: R. Gillon and A. Lloyd (Eds) *Principles of Health Care Ethics*. Chichester: Wiley.

Wing, J.K. (1972) Principles of evaluation. In: J.K. Wing and A.M. Hailey (Eds) *Evaluating Community Psychiatric Service: The Camberwell Register 1964–1971*. London: Oxford University Press.

Wing, J.K. (1978) Medical and social science and medical and social care. In: J. Barnes and N. Connelly (Eds) *Social Care Research*. London: Bedford Square Press.

Wing, J.K. (1986) The cycle of planning and evaluation. In: G. Wilkinson and H. Freeman (Eds) *The Provision of Mental Health Services in Britain: The Way Ahead*. London: Gaskell Press.

Wing, J.K., Cooper, J.E. and Sartorius, N. (1974) *Measurement and Classification of Psychiatric Symptoms: An Instruction Manual for the PSE and CATEGO Program*. Cambridge: Cambridge University Press.

Wykes, T. and Sturt, E. (1986) The measurement of social behaviour in psychiatric patients: an assessment of the reliability and validity of the SBS Schedule. *British Journal of Psychiatry*, **148**, 1–11.

Xenitidis, K., Thornicroft, G., Leese, M., et al. (2000) Reliability and validity of the CANDID – a needs assessment instrument for adults with learning disabilities and mental health problems. *British Journal of Psychiatry*, **176**, 473–478.

Further reading

Allen, D. et al. (1991) *Meeting the Challenge: Some UK Perspectives on Community Services for People with Learning Difficulties and Challenging Behaviour*. London: King's Fund Centre.

Altman, D.G. (1991) *Practical Statistics for Medical Research*. London: Chapman and Hall.

Baldwin, S. (1998) Problems with needs: where theory meets practice in mental health services. In: S. Baldwin (Ed.) *Needs Assessment and Community Care: Clinical Practice and Policy Making*. Oxford: Butterworth-Heinemann.

Ballinger, B.R., Ballinger, C.B., Reid, A.H. and McQueen, E. (1991) The psychiatric symptoms, diagnoses and care needs of 100 mentally handicapped patients. *British Journal of Psychiatry*, **158**, 255–259.

Bouras, N. and Drummond, C. (1992) Behaviour and psychiatric disorders of people with mental handicaps living in the community. *Journal of Intellectual Disability Research*, **36**, 349–357.

Department of Health (1993) *Services for People with Learning Disabilities and Challenging Behaviour or Mental Health Needs* (Chairman: Professor J. Mansell). London: HMSO.

Hester Adrian Research Centre (1994) *Psychiatric Assessment Schedule for Adults with a Developmental Disability, ICD-10 Version.* University of Manchester: Hester Adrian Research Centre.

Holloway, F. (1991) Case management for the mentally ill: looking at the evidence. *International Journal of Social Psychiatry*, **37**, 2–13.

Landis, J.R. and Koch, G.G. (1977) Cited in Altman, D.G. (1991) *Practical Statistics for Medical Research.* London: Chapman and Hall.

Leasage, A.D., Mignolli, G., Faccincani, C. and Tansella, M. (1991) Standardised assessment of the needs for care in a cohort of patients with schizophrenic psychosis. In: Community based psychiatry long-term patterns of care in south-Verona. *Psychological Medicine Monograph Supplement*, **19**, 27–33.

Lightfoot, J. (1995) Identifying needs and setting priorities: issues of theory, policy and practice. *Health and Social Care*, **3**, 105–144.

Lockwood, A. and Marshall, M. (1999) Can a standardised needs assessment be used to improve the care of people with severe mental disorders? A pilot study of 'needs feedback'. *Journal of Advanced Nursing*, **30**, 1408–1415.

Moss, S., Prosser, H., Ibbotson, B. and Goldberg, D. (1996) Respondent and informant accounts of psychiatric symptoms in a sample of patients with learning disability. *Journal of Intellectual Disability Research*, **40**, 457–465.

Patel, P., Goldberg, D. and Moss, S. (1993) Psychiatric morbidity in older people with moderate and severe learning disability: the Prevalence Study. *British Journal of Psychiatry*, **163**, 481–491.

Stevens, A. and Raftery, J. (1994) The stimulus for needs assessment: reforming health services. In: A. Stevens and J. Raftery (Eds) *Health Care Needs Assessment: The Epidemiologically Based Needs Assessment Reviews.* Oxford: Radcliffe Medical Press.

Chapter 6

Learning disability nursing

Learning disability nursing has a long history going back to the history of learning disability itself and the institutional models of care that prevailed during the last two centuries. The question that most people who are not familiar with people with learning disabilities ask is 'What is learning disability nursing?' There are two ways of seeing learning disability nursing within the current context of nursing: one as a specialised professional qualification, which focuses on the principles of enabling an individual to lead an independent healthy life, and the other as a specialised professional nursing qualification subjected to ignorant interpretations. The purpose of this chapter is not to explore the tensions and perceptions of learning disability nursing that prevail in the family of nursing, but to focus on and explore the role of learning disability nursing in the care of people with dual diagnosis from a therapeutic perspective.

Key themes

- The nature of learning disability nursing
- Definitions of learning disability nursing
- Roles of learning disability nurses
- The learning disability nurse as therapist

What is learning disability nursing?

The development of learning disability nursing is embedded within the history of learning disability services based in large institutions. The attempt by doctors to find an organic basis for learning disability in the 19th century played a role in the creation of skilled assistants to care for this population (Dingwall et al. 1988). Until 1919 learning disability nursing (known as *mental deficiency nursing* at that time) was seen as part of mental nursing (Department of Health and Social Security 1979). It is argued that mental deficiency nursing shared many of the characteristics of mental nursing, but differed in one significant aspect

– its emphasis on training to provide long-term care rather than cure. Due to this emphasis, the General Nursing Council (GNC) failed to accept it as a valid branch of nursing as mental deficiency nurses were not seen as carers of the sick but as educators and not 'real' nurses (Mitchell 1998a, 1998b).

Over the last three decades, learning disability nursing has had to adjust to major social policy changes affecting the philosophy of care and practice. Examples include seeing the hospital as a home for people with learning disabilities, as outlined in the Mittler report (DHSS 1978); the closure of long-stay hospitals and move into community settings; continuing change in roles in the context of health and social care provisions; the mixed economy of care; the introduction of care management and care planning. These are some of the key social policy changes that have impacted on the role of the learning disability nurse. As a result, learning disability nursing is constantly under review and adapting to the changing foci and philosophy of care, leading to the development of new roles, skills and methods of working with people with learning disabilities and care providers.

The role of a learning disability nurse was described as one of providing individualised care to people with learning disabilities and their families and collaborating with others to create alternatives to hospital care (Kay et al. 1995). Moulster and Turnbull (2004) argue that the purpose of nursing people with learning disabilities is to work in partnership with the individual to improve his or her personal autonomy. They suggest that this can be achieved by:

- Mitigating the effects of disability
- Achieving optimum health
- Facilitating access to and encouraging involvement in local communities
- Increasing personal competence
- Maximising choice
- Enhancing the contribution of others either formally or informally involved in supporting the individual

The definition of learning disability nursing as identified in the Project 2000 framework for nurse education states that:

'the function of the nurse for people with mental handicap is to directly and skilfully assist the individual and his/her family, whatever the handicap, in the acquisition, development and maintenance of those skills that, given the necessary ability, would be performed unaided and to do this in such a way as to enable independence to be gained as rapidly and as fully as possible in an environment that maintains a quality of life that would be acceptable to fellow citizens of the same age.' (United Kingdom Central Council for Nursing 1987)

This definition, which is an adapted version of the Virginia Henderson (Henderson 1961) definition of nursing, maps out the key areas of the role of the learning disability nurse. It is important to see learning disability nursing with a clear and powerful value base for the provision of care and support through the principles of an *'ordinary life'* (Alaszewski et al. 2001). The lives of people with learning disabilities who experience mental health problems constantly face double stigma (from learning disability and mental health diagnostic labels), resulting in social isolation and barriers in accessing appropriate health and social care services. The key question here is how best to enhance and develop the clinical practice of learning disability nurses working with people with dual diagnosis. We believe that whilst promoting ordinary life, learning disability nurses need to focus on the therapeutic aspect of nursing as identified by McMahon and Pearson (1998) 'as the practice(s) of nursing which have a healing effect or those which result in a movement towards health or wellness' (p. 7). By focusing on the therapeutic nursing role, we do not believe that the value base of an ordinary life will be lost in learning disability nursing practice, and in many ways this may help in exploring and strengthening the therapeutic roles of the learning disability nurse.

Therapeutic nursing

We wish to explore the key therapeutic activities of nursing as identified by McMahon and Pearson (1998) in their work of *Nursing as Therapy*. The rationale for this exploration is based on our belief that the role of the learning disability nurse in the field of dual diagnosis matches that of a nurse as therapist. A key component of therapeutic nursing is the concept of holism, which assumes that the mind and the body are inextricably linked and that an influence on one will lead to change in the other (McMahon 1998). Holism is an important concept in the care of people with learning disabilities, where the person's own perception of the self and the carers' (or the professionals') perceptions of the person (with learning disabilities) are linked to the facilitation of the well-being of the individual.

McMahon (1998) argues that holism puts the emphasis on the nurse empowering the person (or the patient from a medical model) to take responsibility in identifying his or her own goals and using the nurse as a resource in regaining his/her own health. Many people with dual diagnosis may not be able to identify their own goals for well-being without help from a professional whom they know best. Learning disability nurses by nature of their training and experience work closely with individuals and their families and play a key role in the co-ordination of therapeutic care. Too often learning disability nurses get embroiled in the care co-ordination role or in the role of care manager, and not much emphasis is given to the learning disability nurse as a therapist.

A review of learning disability nursing, *Continuing the Commitment* (Kay et al. 1995), highlights that the key roles of learning disability nurses fall in the following areas:

- Assessment of need
- Health surveillance and health promotion
- Developing personal competence
- The use of enhanced therapeutic skills
- Managing and leading teams of staff
- Enhancing the quality of support
- Enablement and empowerment
- Co-ordinating services

In this context, let us explore the therapeutic activities of nursing as identified by McMahon (1998) and examine its relevance to learning disability nursing in the care of people with dual diagnosis.

Developing partnership, intimacy and reciprocity in the nurse–patient relationship

This focuses on the therapeutic interaction with the person, which will influence the reaction and compliance from the person in addressing his or her needs or goals for well-being. Emphasis is placed on the behaviour of the nurse in gaining the trust and confidence of the person, which in turn will be influential in building a climate of partnership and intimacy. The three factors that are crucial in working with a person with dual diagnosis consist of:

- Forming a relationship based on trust, respecting the person's personal integrity regardless of his or her behaviour and/or mental state
- Gaining the confidence of the person through interactions involving personal care and interpersonal interactions, thus promoting physical and psychological safety
- Enabling the person to express his or her thoughts, feelings and emotions using established and imaginative communication patterns

Building a therapeutic relationship is key to understanding the thoughts, feelings and behaviours of the person with dual diagnosis, thus creating a climate of mutual understanding and respect leading to positive growth and emotional well-being. This means that the nurse needs to demonstrate a non-judgemental approach when working with people with dual diagnosis and aim to foster an environment where people can express their thoughts and feelings freely and safely within the Professional Code of Conduct (Nursing and Midwifery Council 2002). Hildegard Peplau's (1952) pioneering work on the therapeutic relationship and its approach to nursing, the one-to-one relationship between nurses and patients, is helpful in putting this into context. According to Peplau:

'the nursing process is educative and therapeutic when the nurse and the patient can come to know and respect each other, as persons who are alike, and yet different, as persons who share in the solution of problems.' (Peplau 1952, p. 9)

The established therapeutic relationship with a person with dual diagnosis enables the learning disability nurse to realise the potentialities and worthiness of the person. Reflection of the relationship – the nature of the person's behaviour and attitude towards the practitioner, the attitudes and behaviours of the nurse practitioner towards the person with dual diagnosis, the reactions of other professionals and service providers towards the person and the nurse practitioner – can contribute to a better understanding of the problems and needs of the person in the light of the value-based relationship.

Caring and comforting

The act of caring and comforting is a complex process, which is more than the general feeling of goodwill towards the person (or the patient). This encompasses the psychological comfort and warmth expressed in the caring for another human being, which rests on the nurse–patient relationship. Through caring and comforting, the learning disability nurse should be able to perceive the person's difficulties in adjusting to his/her environment brought upon by his/her behaviour and mental distress.

The act of caring and comforting helps the assessment process. In therapeutic nursing, assessment is the key in understanding the lifestyle of a person who requires nursing care. Assessment is the process of gathering information using specialised knowledge and skills, and identifying and documenting the person's level of functioning, the presenting problems such as behaviour and mental state and the general needs of the person. In caring for a person with dual diagnosis, a learning disability nurse will have to undertake a range of general assessments to identify general health issues and also specialised assessments to understand the behaviour and mental state of the person.

The positive nature of the therapeutic relationship with the person with dual diagnosis will undoubtedly help the assessment process through the interpretation of complex communication patterns and behaviours, its function and meaning and its relevance in day-to-day caring. The nature and impact of mental illness and its manifestation in people with multiple and profound learning disabilities is an intricate process. As a result, caring and comforting persons with multiple and profound learning disabilities and mental illness requires sharp observational and perceptive skills in recognising their verbal and non-verbal cues and in identifying appropriate responses. This is well stated by Sines (1995) who conceptualised the empowerment model in learning disability practice and suggested that nurses spend a major part of their time engaged in the support and care of people with severe learning disabilities. Through the process of their interaction with people with learning disabilities they are able to acquire both specific and general skills in needs assessment and diagnosis of their clients.

Using evidence-based interventions

The use of evidence-based practice and practice-based evidence is crucial in developing nursing practice for people with learning disabilities. The lack of a professional knowledge base of learning disability nursing in the care of people with dual diagnosis makes it difficult for nurses to articulate the nature of the nursing contribution and its effectiveness. Too often learning disability nursing relies on a knowledge base that is drawn from other disciplines such as psychiatry, psychology, sociology and education.

From historical accounts and published literature we can see that learning disability nurses have made a significant contribution to the care and welfare of people with learning disabilities and their carers. Alaszewski et al.'s report (2001) on the changing roles and education of learning disability nurses highlights many examples of their contribution to helping people with learning disability, including:

- The possession of specialist and integrated knowledge of people with learning disabilities and its impact in multidisciplinary teamwork
- The perception of the family – the role of the learning disability nurse as a friend

There is a need to develop a well-documented knowledge (or evidence) base for learning disability nursing in order to strengthen its professional identity and to enhance its growth reflecting the holistic care spectrum. Sines (1995) argues that much of the knowledge acquired by learning disability nurses has been acquired from the intimacy of their relationship with people with learning disabilities over a considerable period of time. For example, learning disability nurses are able to form therapeutic relationships with people with dual diagnosis and are able to identify the nature and manifestation of mental illness through their close working relationships. Sines (1995) suggests that this form of knowledge acquisition involves the capacity to avoid introspection and to share findings with others (both within and outside the nursing profession) with the aim of validating and confirming the information about a client's needs and requirements. Sines calls this aesthetic knowledge, which is considered to be a central element in learning disability care because it refers to the dynamic nature of nursing practice itself, or in other words this could be considered to be practice-based evidence.

A systematic account of practice-based evidence is crucial in the development of a knowledge base for learning disability nursing. Peplau (1988) proposes development of a practice-based theory and urges nurses to use nursing situations as a source of observations from which unique nursing concepts could be derived. This emphasises the need for learning disability nurses to understand, internalise and act upon the general principles gained from experiential learning. Moulster and Turnbull (2004) take up the theme of generating knowledge from practice:

'if the aim of learning disability nursing is to help individuals with learning disabilities to construct a vision of the future, then this vision is more likely to be realised if the nurse is able to generate good quality information and knowledge from their encounter with the individual.' (p. 67)

A practice-based evidence or knowledge base for learning disability nursing in the care of people with dual diagnosis can only be initiated through the reflection of nurses' therapeutic experiences. This should include:

- Their experience of conducting assessments and the personalised approaches adopted to facilitate the assessment process.
- Their experience of planning care within the multidisciplinary team, taking into account the nature of the person, the place where he or she lives, the impact of care on other people with learning disabilities in the environment, the targeting of resources and planning individualised approaches.
- The rationale and methods used for the intervention or care plans.
- Their first-hand experience of implementing the intervention strategies, the role of the therapeutic relationship during this process, shaping and adapting the intervention strategies to suit the individual and the context of that person, as well as the positive and negative consequences of interventions for the individual, carers and other people involved.
- Their experience of constant monitoring of the interventions.
- Their experience of the problems and dilemmas encountered in partnership working and the solutions adopted for strengthening partnership working.

McMahon (1998) suggests that practitioners should govern the direction of knowledge development in the future. Hence, in generating a practice-based evidence or practice-based knowledge learning disability nurses need to reflect on and document their actions aimed at the well-being of people with dual diagnosis.

Teaching

Teaching people to improve their healthy lifestyles is an essential part of therapeutic nursing. This is an area that is not congruent with the traditional forms of nursing as they lay heavy emphasis on the model of caring for the sick person. However, in learning disability nursing the development of personal competence through teaching and empowerment is seen as an integral part of nursing practice. The *Continuing the Commitment* document (Kay et al. 1995) states that a significant part of the role of the nurse involves helping people with learning disability to acquire skills that will increase their competence and feelings of control. Helping people to acquire skills of self-care, personal control, management of feelings and emotions such as anger and anxiety are pillars of therapeutic nursing activities with people with learning disabilities.

The role of teaching and facilitating the acquisition and development of skills is not confined to work with people with learning disabilities. In nursing practice the facilitation of therapeutic care depends on having a knowledgeable and skilled team of practitioners and helpers. The therapeutic care for people with dual diagnosis is delivered in a range of settings such the person's own home, in mainstream mental health services, in group homes, in specialist units designed to facilitate and monitor assessment and treatment and in secure provisions. How can we plan and deliver consistent care approaches in a range of settings through team and partnership working? This is a complex process that requires good understanding of the knowledge base of dual diagnosis, expertise in assessment and interventions, good leadership and teamworking skills, efficient and effective communication skills and ability to reflect on practice and personal experiences. Learning disability nurses need to play an effective role in the development of the therapeutic team through the facilitation of knowledge and skills across the team, through positive monitoring of the performance of team members and through clinical supervision.

Manipulating the environment

This focuses on the creation of a therapeutic environment, which can be interpreted to mean the interpersonal as well as the physical environment (McMahon 1998). Over the years, learning disability nursing has moved away from care focused on physical environments (hospitals) to a system of care that meets people's needs, in whatever environments they live. The advocacy and empowerment movement and the articulation by people with learning disabilities themselves of the need to be treated as *people* with equal rights just like any other citizens have led to the conceptualisation and creation of inclusive services. O'Brien and Lyle (1987) list five accomplishments (choice, relationships, dignity and esteem, participation and integration, and competence) that have played a crucial role in shaping the creation of inclusive mainstream services.

Many people with learning disabilities live in purpose-built residential environments such as group homes, residential homes or nursing homes depending on the kind of help and support required for day-to-day living and their health needs. The majority of people with dual diagnosis tend to use specialist services within learning disability services (such as specially staffed group homes, assessment and treatment units, medium secure and secure provisions). The environment in which care is planned and delivered needs to take into account the environmental influences shaping a person's identity. An environment that is threatening or controlling is not part of therapeutic care, as this eats into a person's self-respect and esteem. As a result care needs to be delivered in an environment that enhances the skills and abilities of the person with dual diagnosis and that observes and promotes the key principles of rights, independence, choice and inclusion as identified in the White Paper *Valuing People* (Department of Health 2001).

Management of these environments is a role normally taken by learning disability nurses and this requires knowledge and skills in the deployment of staff and an understanding of the skills mix required for organising and delivering effective therapeutic care.

Facing the future

Research into the changing roles and education of learning disability nurses (Alaszewski et al. 2001) highlights the overlapping roles of the learning disability nurse with other members of the multidisciplinary team. Alaszewski et al.'s research report states that:

'Nurses saw their role in terms of providing direct care, integrating the team and providing specialist knowledge. They (learning disability nurses) combined the knowledge and understanding of the needs of people with learning disabilities and knowledge of the needs and care of specific individuals.'

The discussion on the role of the learning disability nurse as a therapist working with people with dual diagnosis has highlighted the need to develop a knowledge base that will reflect contemporary nursing practice. Learning disability nurses need to emphasise their knowledge base, clinical skills and working practices in a range of settings in terms of the assessment and the utilisation of systematic processes in the identification of individual needs and in the planning of person-centred care. The key components of person-centred care as identified by Talerico (2003) consist of:

- Knowing the person as an individual and being responsive to individual and family characteristics
- Providing care that is meaningful to the person in ways that reflect the individual's values, preferences and needs
- Viewing care recipients as biopsychosocial human beings
- Fostering development of consistent and trusting care-giving relationships
- Emphasising freedom of choice and individually defined, reasonable risk taking
- Promoting physical and emotional comfort
- Appropriately involving the person's family, friends and social network

Learning disability nurses are incorporating these principles into the care of people with dual diagnosis.

Developing a future workforce

Meeting the needs of people within the community who have learning disabilities and exhibit challenging behaviour and who may have an associated mental health problem raises particular policy questions. The provision of effective community services for people with this particular combination of complex needs requires a skilled workforce. Jukes and O'Shea (1998) express concerns relating to nurse education and training with regard to the implications for practice surrounding diagnosis across cultures, classification of illness, and the status and influence of psychological assessments within the field of mental health and learning disability. They emphasise the concept of empowerment and recognise that if a person's needs are to be adequately addressed, community mental health and learning disability nurses must make dynamic alliances with communities. This will redirect the power relationship to the community and subsequently respond to the demands for cultural diversity sensitively from within health care provision and services.

Naylor and Clifton (1993) undertook a study to investigate definitions of challenging behaviour and mental health problems in relation to people with learning disabilities, therapeutic interventions for meeting these needs, models of service provision for such people and the implications for developing a skilled workforce to meet this particular combination of needs. The study's findings suggest that definitions of challenging behaviour are varied and the diagnosis of mental illness in people with learning disabilities appears to be more poorly developed in the UK than in the USA. Those whose needs include both learning disability and mental health problems are at risk of losing out in the provision of services for either category. There are two differing models of service provision for people with these needs – the 'campus' model and the 'ordinary life' model. There are considerable tensions between the two approaches. Professional tensions with regard to both therapeutic responses and service models must be resolved if people with this particular combination of complex needs are to receive a comprehensive, needs-led service provided by an appropriately skilled workforce.

It has been suggested that learning disability nursing has a central role to play in the promotion of mental health for people with learning disabilities (Department of Health 1995). However, learning disability nursing presently operates without a clear model of mental health. Therefore, before this potential can be realised there is a need to establish the common ground between the discourses of learning disability nursing and those of psychiatric nursing that might be related to this client group. Gilbert et al. (1998) propose that an applied behavioural approach has the potential to provide a coherent theory that can link the discourses of normalisation, developmental psychiatry and mental health nursing, whilst also establishing the applied behavioural approach as a powerful technology upon which meaningful interventions can be designed.

Whilst searching for different models of learning disability nursing, it is important that we do not forget the contribution of the learning disability nurse in assessment, interventions and service co-coordination processes for people with dual diagnosis. Aspiring for an ordinary life for people with learning disabilities with mental health needs is a goal that all professionals in all services should work for, but this does not mean that we no longer require nurses specialised in working with people with learning disabilities. Family carers, professionals and support workers often talk about the traumatic experiences of people with learning disabilities in accessing mainstream health services and their marginalised treatment. The same can also be said of people with learning disabilities accessing and using mainstream mental health services in terms of the ignorance of learning disability expressed by some mental health nurses and general psychiatrists. Thus it is vital that there should be trained nurses specialising in learning disabilities who are able to provide the much needed help and support for people with learning disabilities and their carers in combating health inequalities. The planning of a future workforce involving people with learning disabilities should be addressed urgently if these people are to access and receive effective support and care from main-stream health and social care services.

Nursing contribution

Kay et al. (1995) suggest that 'one of the best ways of articulating the contribu-tion of any professional is through the demonstration of positive outcomes for people with learning disabilities' (p. 38). Learning disability nurses supporting people with dual diagnosis in residential, in-patient and outreach services should be able to articulate their positive contribution to health improvements, for example in:

- The assessment process which may include the overall level of functioning of the person using standardised tools, specific assessments of behaviour and mental state along with the psychiatrist, functional analysis of behavi-ours and risk assessments.
- Planning of psychosocial and nursing interventions, the care planning process, day-to-day adaptations to the implantation of these interventions, helping models to be carried out and the outcome of these interventions.
- Overall evaluation of the interventions, specific nursing initiatives and approaches that may have contributed to a positive outcome.
- Planning future care for the person in terms of help and support required, environmental aspects, safety and security.

Learning disability nurses need to work with nurses in other settings such as the acute ward in a mainstream mental health service. In this context, it is important to value the contribution of mental health nurses in the well-being of the person and to work in partnership with mental health colleagues in planning appropriate care and services.

Conclusion

In this chapter we have explored the role of the learning disability nurse as a therapist in caring for people with dual diagnosis. The contribution of learning disability nursing as a specialist form of nursing was considered in describing the distinct roles of the learning disability nurse. The policy changes in health and social care have had a major impact on the working of learning disability nurses and their positive contribution in direct care, the co-ordination of care and liaison activities needs to be better articulated.

References

Alaszewski, A., Gates, B., Motherby, E., Manthorpe, J. and Ayer, S. (2001) *Educational Preparation for Learning Disability Nursing: Outcomes Evaluation of the Contribution of Learning Disability Nurses Within the Multi-professional, Multi-agency Team*. London: English National Board.

Department of Health (1995) *The Health of the Nation: A Strategy for People with Learning Disabilities*. London: HMSO.

Department of Health (2001) *Valuing People: A New Strategy for Learning Disability for the 21st Century*. London: The Stationery Office.

Department of Health and Social Security (DHSS) (1978) *Helping Mentally Handicapped People in Hospital. A Report to the Secretary of State for Health and Social Services by the National Development Group for the Mentally Handicapped* (Chairman: P. Mittler). London: HMSO.

Department of Health and Social Security (DHSS) (1979) *Report of the Committee of Inquiry into Mental Handicap Nursing and Care*. Vols I and II, Cmnd 7468-I, 7468-II, (Chairman: Mrs. P. Jay). London: HMSO.

Dingwall, R., Rafferty, A.M. and Webster, C. (1988) *An Introduction to the Social History of Nursing*. London: Routledge.

Gilbert, T., Todd, M. and Jackson, N. (1998) People with learning disabilities who also have mental health problems: practice issues and directions for learning disability nursing. *Journal of Advanced Nursing*, **27**, 1151–1157.

Henderson, V. (1961) *Nature of Nursing*. Mosby: St Louis.

Jukes, M. and O'Shea, K. (1998) Transcultural therapy 2: mental health and learning disability. *British Journal of Nursing*, **7**, 1268–1272.

Kay, B., Rose, S. and Turnbull, J. (1995) *Continuing the Commitment: Report of the Learning Disability Nursing Project*. London: HMSO.

McMahon, R. (1998) Therapeutic nursing: theory, issues and practice. In: R. McMahon and A. Pearson (Eds) *Nursing as Therapy*. Cheltenham: Stanley Thornes.

McMahon, R. and Pearson, A. (1998) *Nursing as Therapy*, 2nd edition. Cheltenham: Stanley Thornes.

Mitchell, D. (1998a) The origins of learning disability nursing. *International History of Nursing Journal*, **4**, 10–16.

Mitchell, D. (1998b) In a league of their own. *Nursing Times*, **94** (10), 30–31.

Moulster, G. and Turnbull, J. (2004) The purpose and practice of learning disability nursing. In: J. Turnbull (Ed.) *Learning Disability Nursing*. Oxford: Blackwell Science.

Naylor, V. and Clifton, M. (1993) People with learning disabilities – meeting complex needs. *Health and Social Care in the Community*, **1**, 343–353.

Nursing and Midwifery Council (2002) *Professional Code of Conduct*. London: NMC.

O'Brien, J. and Lyle, C. (1987) *Framework for Accomplishment*. Georgia: GA Responsive Service Systems Associates.

Peplau, H.E. (1952) *Interpersonal Relations in Nursing*. New York: Putnam.

Peplau, H.E. (1988) The art and science of nursing: similarities: differences and relations. *Nursing Science Quarterly*, **1**, 8–15.

Sines, D. (1995) Impaired autonomy – the challenge of caring. *Journal of Clinical Nursing*, **4**, 109–115.

Talerico, K.A. (2003) Person centred care: an important approach for the 21st century health care. *Journal of Psychosocial Nursing*, **41**, 12–16.

United Kingdom Central Council for Nursing (1987) *Project 2000: Working Papers and Final Report*. London: UKCC.

Chapter 7

Psychopharmacological approaches and ECT

The use of medication, its effectiveness in people with dual diagnosis and the consequences of its use in terms of side effects are contentious issues. It is essential for nurses to have a broad understanding of psychopharmacology and its effectiveness in people with dual diagnosis. This chapter aims to provide such an understanding, discusses the role of psychopharmacology in the treatment of mental illness, types of medication and good practice in the prescription of medication for people with dual diagnosis.

Key themes

- Exploration of the various types of medication
- Examination of the side effects of medication
- Highlighting good practice guidelines

Psychopharmacology and people with learning disability

Psychopharmacology is the term used to describe the study of the effects of drugs upon mental functions and illness. Drugs that affect psychiatric conditions are called psychotropic (affecting the mind) drugs. Broadly, psychotropic drugs are classified according to their main therapeutic use: antidepressants; antipsychotics (also known as neuroleptics or major tranquillisers); hypnotics and anxiolytics; mood stabilisers; stimulants; antidementia drugs; antiparkinsonian drugs; and anti-epileptic drugs.

People with learning disabilities are more likely to suffer from mental illness than other people. Pooled results of studies suggest that 2 to 6% of the population have schizophrenia and 3 to 8% have affective disorders. About half of those in hospital have neuroses or behaviour disorders such as hyperkinesis, autism, hysteria or anxiety states and about 25 to 40% have epilepsy (Cookson et al. 2002). Thus people with learning disabilities are one of the most highly medicated populations in our society. The Royal College of Psychiatrists has published guidelines on the use of high doses of antipsychotic (neuroleptic) medication following concern in the media about sudden deaths associated with such drugs (Thompson 1994). It is estimated that between 20 and 45% of people with learning disability are on antipsychotic drugs, 14 to 30% of whom are on such drugs to manage challenging behaviour (Deb and Fraser 1994). In fact the most common reason for prescribing antipsychotic medication to people with learning disability is not psychosis but the management of behaviour problems (Molyneaux et al. 2000). Clarke et al. (1990) reported that 36% of patients in three different residential settings were on psychotropic medication without a formal psychiatric diagnosis. Although the use of such medication in the treatment of psychiatric disorders can be justified, its use in the management of behaviour disorders alone is more controversial.

Prescribing for people with learning disabilities can be problematic for various reasons. First, there is the difficulty in arriving at an accurate diagnosis due to communication deficits and atypical behavioural features of mental disorder especially in those with more severe or profound disability. For the same reasons self report of adverse effects is less likely. Abnormal physical movements are frequent in this population and therefore movement disorders such as tardive dyskinesia or akathisia (excessive restlessness) may be more difficult to identify as a side effect of antipsychotic medication. Thus such side effects may be missed, underdetected or mistaken for challenging behaviour and may result in a further harmful increase in the dose of the medication. Similarly toxic effects of antiepileptic drugs or lithium, for example slurred speech, drowsiness, confusion and ataxia (drunken gait), may be thought of as being due to the learning disability itself, the so-called diagnostic overshadowing effect. Parkinsonian side effects from the use of antipsychotic drugs can lead to stiffness and shakiness, further impairing the already limited mobility in those with physical handicaps or cerebral palsy. Another important and serious side effect of long-term exposure to antipsychotic medication is tardive dyskinesia (see discussion later in this chapter).

It is important to remember that drug treatment is one of many strategies used to manage mental disorder, especially behaviour disorders. A comprehensive multidisciplinary assessment and formulation of an individualised care plan is important. The overall aim of the treatment is not only to control symptoms but also to provide a better quality of life for people with learning disability and their carers. Drug treatment aimed at a specific psychiatric disorder such as schizophrenia or depression is justified and its efficacy should ideally be assessed by ongoing monitoring of specified target symptoms, for example low mood, sleep disturbance, panic attacks, change in appetite or weight, outbursts of anger and so on. Treatment should be based on evidence of effectiveness as far as possible and in the UK such evidence-based guidelines are increasingly provided by organisations such as the National Institute of Clinical Excellence (NICE) and the British Association of Psychopharmacology. In the field of learning disability, Reiss and Aman (1997) invited 115 scientists, practitioners and consumers from 11 nations to form an international consensus panel on best practices and the clinical benefits of psychoactive medicines in those with intellectual or learning disability. In the introduction to the paper based on this panel's deliberation, they comment that very little scientific research has been reported regarding the safety and efficacy of the use of psychotropic medicines in people with intellectual or learning disability. Thus the use of such drugs is often based on extrapolation of knowledge regarding their effects on people who do not have learning disability. They find this a questionable basis for practice. Responses to drugs may be altered by an abnormality or damage to the brain's structure, and hence side effects may readily appear. Barbiturates especially may make the person irritable; thus phenobarbitone and primidone are unsuitable as antiepileptics in people with learning disabilities. Benzodiazepines such as diazepam and lorazepam can cause disinhibition and irritability in those with organic brain impairment. One also needs to keep in mind the possibility of drug interactions especially with antiepileptic drugs, which are commonly prescribed in this population. Polypharmacy (that is using multiple drugs often belonging to the same class, for example using two to three antipsychotic drugs together) and overmedication (using doses that are too high) can lead to excessive sedation and tiredness, further impairing the person's quality of life. Furthermore the person with learning disability may be unable to recognise and report on side effects associated with such medication. The occurrence and frequency of side effects in people with learning disability have received little systematic study so far.

Good practice in prescribing psychotropic medication

The following guidelines it is hoped will enable more informed and rational use of psychotropic medication:

- Use psychotropic medication after multidisciplinary discussion of potential risks and benefits and agreement that it is in the person's best interests, especially when the individual is unable to give informed consent.
- Use should be based on a psychiatric diagnosis or specific behavioural–pharmacologic hypothesis after a comprehensive diagnostic formulation and/or functional behavioural analysis.
- Assess capacity to give informed consent. Informed consent may be difficult to obtain from a person with learning disability, and therefore active consultation with carers is important. Carers should be given adequate information about the reasons for using specific medication and the potential side effects, and frank discussion about lack of evidence base when used for behavioural problems is helpful.
- Measure treatment efficacy by objectively defining index behaviours and quality-of-life outcomes.
- Monitor side effects using appropriate assessment instruments when possible.
- Use lowest optimum dose. Avoid frequent drug or dose changes. Avoid use of high dose antipsychotic drugs for long periods without evaluation.

Withdraw medication when it is not beneficial or is causing serious adverse effects.

- Monitor clinical practice via audit through peer or external quality review.
- Do not use for convenience, as substitute for psychosocial services or in quantities that interfere with quality of life.
- Avoid long-term use of benzodiazepines whenever possible.

Types of psychotropic medication, indications and side effects

Antipsychotic medication

Antipsychotic drugs are thought to act by interfering with dopaminergic transmission in the brain, particularly by blockage of dopamine D2 receptors. They also have an effect on other receptors, for example serotonergic, histaminergic, cholinergic and alpha-adrenergic receptors. Antipsychotics are usually divided into two classes: the older 'typical' agents, such as chlorpromazine and haloperidol, and the newer 'atypical' agents. The difference between the two is mainly to do with the reduced risk with atypical agents of extrapyramidal side effects (EPSE) and less elevation of the hormone prolactin. The *British National Formulary* (BNF) (2004) currently lists amisulpride (Solian), olanzapine (Zyprexa), quetiapine (seroquel), risperidone (Risperdal), sertindole (Serdolect), aripiprazole (Abilify) and zotepine (Zoleptil) as atypical antipsychotics. Due to ongoing concerns about cardiac side effects, sertindole is only available for use direct from the manufacturers and ongoing cardiac monitoring is a prerequisite for its use. Clozapine (Clozaril) is also listed in the BNF as an atypical antipsychotic. Its use is restricted to individuals with schizophrenia who are unresponsive or intolerant to 'conventional' antipsychotic therapy.

'Typical' or 'traditional' antipsychotics

These include the so-called older antipsychotic drugs, for example haloperidol, chlorpromazine, trifluoperazine, thioridazine, pimozide and sulpiride. Chlorpromazine (Largactil) was the first antipsychotic drug to be used in psychiatry in 1952. This drug belongs to the group of phenothiazines. Within the general population, chlorpromazine has been used for the treatment of schizophrenia and other psychosis; mania, control of the violent patient, insomnia, tension, anxiety and agitation; nausea and vomiting and appetite stimulation in anorexia nervosa. It is thought that patients with brain damage may be unusually sensitive to phenothiazines. The tendency to have fits may be slightly increased in epilepsy, but these drugs are useful for controlling the irritability and aggression that sometimes occur in epilepsy. For acutely disturbed states, chlorpromazine has a prolonged calming effect without impairment of consciousness (Cookson et al. 2002). It is useful in the treatment of schizophrenia, particularly the paranoid and catatonic subtypes. Thioridazine (Melleril) is another typical drug belonging to the phenothiazine group. At one time thioridazine was widely used to control behavioural disturbance in people with learning disability and those with dementia. After reports of excess deaths of people on this drug, mainly elderly people, its use has become more restricted. It is now indicated for second-line treatment of schizophrenia under specialist supervision and due to its potential to cause fatal cardiac arrhythmias, an ECG should be carried out before starting and after any dose increase. In a person with learning disability with a clear psychiatric diagnosis, for example schizophrenia or mania, the principles of using antipsychotic drugs are similar to those in the general population. However, a recent Cochrane review of the use of antipsychotic medication for schizophrenia in people with learning disability (Duggan and Brylewski 1999) found only one relevant randomised trial that included four people with a dual diagnosis of schizophrenia and learning disability. The reviewers concluded that there was 'no trial evidence at present to guide the use of antipsychotic medication for those with both learning disability and schizophrenia and there was an urgent need for more randomized trials of good quality in this population'. The same authors conducted another Cochrane systematic review (Brylewski and Duggan 1998) to determine the effectiveness of antipsychotic medication for people with learning disability and challenging behaviour. They found only three randomised trials of satisfactory quality. These provided 'no evidence of whether antipsychotic medication helps or harms adults with learning disability and challenging behaviour'.

Important side effects of antipsychotic medication

All antipsychotic agents have associated side effects (Box 7.1). These may include extrapyramidal side effects, for example parkinsonism (tremor, muscle stiffness, shakiness) which may occur gradually; acute dystonic reactions (severe, often painful spasm of muscle groups) which may appear after only a few doses; akathisia (restless legs) and tardive dyskinesia. (abnormal involuntary movements); autonomic effects, such as blurring of vision, glaucoma (abnormally high pressure in the eye), dry mouth and eyes, constipation and difficulty in passing urine with urinary retention; increased prolactin levels (sexual dysfunction, menstrual irregularity); seizures; sedation and weight gain. Cardiac problems with increased risk of ventricular arrhythmias is also important, particularly with thioridazine and sertindole. Antipsychotic drugs may take several weeks to control symptoms and the minimum effective dose possible should be used (NICE 2002).

Extrapyramidal side effects

Acute dystonia

Dystonia is a distortion of posture caused by involuntary contraction of one or more muscle groups. It can be painful and very frightening and can start within hours of taking the medication. It can present as muscle spasm in any

Box 7.1   Side effects of antipsychotic drugs.

- Extrapyramidal side effects (acute dystonia, parkinsonism, akathisia, tardive dyskinesia) are the most troublesome with typical antipsychotics.
- Sedation and lethargy.
- Orthostatic hypotension (fall in blood pressure) on standing and interference with temperature regulation are dose-related and can lead to dizziness and falls.
- Cardiovascular symptoms such as fall in blood pressure, raised heart rate and arrhythmias can occur. Cases of sudden death have been reported.
- Anticholinergic effects include dry mouth, constipation and blurred vision.
- Lowered seizure threshold can lead to seizures (fits).
- Endocrine effects due to raised prolactin levels are associated with menstrual disturbances, amenorrhoea, sexual dysfunction with difficulties achieving erection or orgasm, risk of reduced fertility, increased risk of osteoporosis, secretion of milk from breasts or enlargement of the breasts in men.
- Weight gain.
- Nausea, vomiting, gastric reflux.
- Photosensitivity (liability to sunburn usually at higher drug doses).
- Blood dyscrasias such as agranulocytosis (severe acute reduction of certain blood cells) or leukopenia (reduced number of white cells in the blood).
- Jaundice with phenothiazines. Stop drug.
- Very rarely neuroleptic malignant syndrome (NMS).

part of the body, for example eyes rolling up, head and neck twisted to the side, person may be unable to speak clearly or swallow; in extreme cases the back may arch or the jaw dislocate. Oculogyric crisis can occur with the eyeballs moving up, resulting in difficulty in seeing. The symptoms can appear so bizarre that they can be mistaken for hysteria and often result in the person seeking urgent treatment at A&E. The condition can be reversed quickly by an injection of procyclidine. It occurs early in the course of treatment sometimes after the first dose. Dystonia occurs in about 10% of those prescribed antipsychotic medication. It is more common in young men and those who are neuroleptic-naïve, i.e. those who have not been previously exposed to such drugs. Dystonia is more common with high potency drugs such as haloperidol and appears to be rarer in the elderly.

Parkinsonism

The key features here are: tremor and/or rigidity, reduced facial expression, slow body movements with a stooped stiff posture and shuffling gait, inability to initiate movements, slowed thinking and excess salivation. It occurs in about 20% of those prescribed antipsychotic medication. Elderly females and those with pre-existing neurological or brain damage are at increased risk, for example owing to a stroke or head injury. Parkinsonism as a side effect usually develops within days or weeks of starting the drug or increasing the dose.

Akathisia

This is characterised by unpleasant inner restlessness with a strong compulsion to move, with foot stamping when seated or constantly crossing/uncrossing legs or pacing up and down. This side effect is so unpleasant that it can occasionally result in suicidal attempts and aggression towards others. It occurs in approximately 25% of those on antipsychotic medication and develops within hours to weeks of starting treatment.

Tardive dyskinesia

One important and serious side effect of long-term exposure to antipsychotic medication is tardive dyskinesia. This is a persistent, sometimes permanent, involuntary movement disorder characterised by smacking of the lips, grimacing, tongue protrusion, grunting, blinking of the eyelids and less commonly involuntary movements of the limbs and trunk. Rarely tardive dyskinesia can affect the larynx or voice box, making the speech slurred. It can also affect the oesophagus or gullet, causing difficulty in swallowing – a problem that can lead to choking on food, particularly in those with severe physical handicaps. Old age, brain damage and female gender appear to be important risk factors in its development. Tardive dyskinesia occurs in 2.5 to 5% of patients per year during long-term treatment. In the elderly 10% or more develop this condition within one year of treatment and up to 40% of patients with schizophrenia over the age of 65 have tardive dyskinesia.

People with learning disability may be more vulnerable to developing side effects with normal doses of medication (Matson et al. 2000). Thus it is important to start with a low dose and increase the dose slowly after careful assessment unlike the practice of starting with a higher dose that is more common in the general population especially in more acute situations. The case example of Simon illustrates tardive dyskinesia.

> Simon was treated in the past with low doses of thioridazine, chlorpromazine and haloperidol. The clinical diagnosis was chronic schizophrenia. He developed EPSE with tremors and cogwheel rigidity on traditional antipsychotics. As the dose of these reduced, he developed abnormal involuntary movements in both upper limbs and the mouth area. The neurologist diagnosed tardive dyskinesia and suggested quetiapine, a new atypical antipsychotic. Simon is doing well on 750 mg daily, with 5 mg diazepam as required for excess anxiety. The abnormal movements have stopped on quetiapine.

Neuroleptic malignant syndrome

This is an extremely rare but potentially fatal side effect. It usually occurs at the initiation of treatment with a high-potency agent but may occur with any of the typical (or atypical agents) at any point. Immediate discontinuation of the medication is essential. Characteristic symptoms include fever, rigidity, confusion, sweating, changing levels of consciousness, fluctuating blood pressure, raised heart rate and swallowing and breathing difficulty. Blood tests show raised levels of creatinine phosphokinase (CPK), a muscle enzyme, high white blood cell count and low serum iron. It occurs in less than 1% of those treated with conventional antipsychotics. The incidence with newer atypical drugs is not known. It has been reported to result in mortality in up to 20% of cases. The following case example of Lorna illustrates neuroleptic malignant syndrome.

Lorna is a 28-year-old woman with moderate learning disability. Her illness started at age 20 with onset of challenging behaviour. Her parents were unable to cope and this led to her admission to a local mentally handicapped hospital. This admission lasted two years and resulted in a diagnosis of bipolar affective disorder (manic depression) in addition to the learning disability. She responded to a combination of antipsychotic medication (clopixol injections) and lithium mood stabiliser. She had two more relapses subsequently. When manic, her behaviour worsened considerably. She would throw things down the toilet, for example toilet rolls, soap dishes, flannels and toothbrushes. She would hit both staff and residents, pinch, spit, throw objects, tear her clothes, bang on the walls, refuse to co-operate, shout, stick her tongue out, repeatedly pull up her socks, rock herself, kick, cough loudly, burp and poke others in the eye. Her concentration span would noticeably deteriorate and she would no longer take an interest in tasks she enjoyed. Over a period of time she unfortunately developed tardive dyskinesia which led to the dose of the clopixol injections being gradually reduced. Initially on dose reduction her mood, behaviour and concentration remained stable. However, she became acutely physically unwell over a period of a month, requiring admission to the medical assessment unit. She developed a high fever with muscle stiffness and confusion. A neurologist diagnosed neuroleptic malignant syndrome. Despite medical treatment her health deteriorated fast and sadly she died in hospital.

Known risk factors for neuroleptic malignant syndrome: Known risk factors include use of high potency typical antipsychotic drugs, rapid increase or rapid decrease in dose, abrupt withdrawal of anticholinergic mediction (e.g. procyclidine), associated physical illness and catatonic features such as violent excitement or stupor. It is vital to stop the antipsychotic drug immediately when side effects occur. Usually urgent treatment by a physician is needed in intensive care. A different class of antipsychotic may be given after full recovery.

Side effects of atypical antipsychotics

Side effects include weight gain, dizziness, postural hypotension (especially during initial dose titration) which may lead to fainting and raised heart rate in some, rarely extrapyramidal symptoms (usually mild and transient, responding to dose reduction or to antimuscarinic drugs), rarely tardive dyskinesia and very rarely neuroleptic malignant syndrome.

Note: Risk of drug-induced arrhythmia and sudden cardiac death is very small with the new drugs. Of much greater concern are other risk factors such as metabolic syndrome, obesity and impaired glucose tolerance leading to diabetes.

Atypical newer antipsychotics

Risperidone (Risperdal)

Risperidone, introduced in 1993, is a benzisoxazole. It is a potent blocker of serotonin (5-HT-2A) and dopamine (D2) receptors. The optimal dose range is 2 to 4 mg twice daily. Doses above 10 mg have no additional benefit but increase the risk of EPS. Doses of more than 16 mg should not be used. Adverse effects of postural hypotension with dizziness and mild sedation can be avoided by increasing the dose gradually. It blocks the D2 receptors in the pituitary and increases prolactin levels to a slightly greater extent than haloperidol. There is a correlation between raised prolactin levels and sexual dysfunction including reduced libido (Cookson et al. 2002). It causes moderate weight gain which is greater than with haloperidol but less than with clozapine and olanzapine. Risperidone is now also available as a long-acting intramuscular injection – a dose of up to 50 mg can be given as an aqueous suspension, every 2 weeks.

Amisulpride (Solian)

Amisulpride, introduced in 1998, is a substituted benzamide. It blocks D2 and D3 dopaminergic receptors, but not D1, D4 or D5 or cholinergic, serotononergic, histaminic or adrenergic receptors. Common adverse effects (in 5 to 10% of cases) include insomnia, anxiety and agitation. Less common side effects (1 to 5%) include somnolence and gastrointestinal effects such as nausea, vomiting and constipation. At doses of 50 to 300 mg it seems to improve the negative symptoms of schizophrenia. At doses above 800 mg it can lead to EPS and raised prolactin levels. The latter can manifest as galactorrhoea and amenorrhoea. Although ECG changes have not been seen at therapeutic doses, overdoses have led to fatal ventricular fibrillation (Cookson et al. 2002).

Olanzapine (Zyprexa)

Olanzapine is a thienobenzodiazepine introduced in 1996. It has potent affinity for dopamine (D1 to D4) receptors as well as serotonin, acetylcholine, noradrenaline (alpha-1) and histamine (H1) receptors. The licensed maximum dose is 20 mg daily. The most common side effects are increased appetite, weight gain, drowsiness and occasionally dry mouth. EPS can occur at doses above 20 mg daily. It can lead to a change in glucose tolerance with raised levels of blood glucose, raised lipids and diabetes, sometimes even in the absence of obesity.

Quetiapine (Seroquel)

Quetiapine is a benzothiazepine introduced in 1997. It binds most strongly to noradrenaline (alpha-1), serotonin (5-HT-2A), acetylcholine (M1), histamine (H1) and dopamine (D2 and D3) receptors. It is a moderately sedative antipsychotic with a very low incidence of acute EPS and is generally well tolerated. The main adverse effects are drowsiness and dyspepsia at high doses, postural hypotension, headache, dry mouth and constipation. Interestingly, sedation with quetiapine is *not* dose dependent. Nasal congestion is occasionally a problem. It does not raise prolactin levels. Weight gain is more comparable to that with haloperidol in the short term, but over months of treatment it is less liable to cause weight gain than olanzapine or clozapine (Cookson et al. 2002). The maximum dose is 800 mg per day. EPS side effects are comparable to placebo at all dose ranges.

Clozapine (Clozaril)

Clozapine is a dibenzodiazepine first produced in 1959. It carries a risk of agranulocytosis (life threatening severe reduction in blood neutrophil counts) in up to 3% of those treated, but this is greatly reduced to about 0.6% if weekly blood counts are performed. The peak rate of agranulocytosis with clozapine occurs at between 4 and 18 weeks, and then falls off sharply. It can only be used orally and the patient must agree to weekly blood counts for 18 weeks, then every 2 weeks until one year, then monthly as long as the treatment continues. Treatment is monitored in the UK by the Clozaril Patient Monitoring Service (CPMS) with which the doctor and pharmacist must register the patient before the pharmacy can dispense it. Clozapine reduces the seizure threshold, which is important in those with epilepsy. It causes seizures in a dose dependent manner – 2% in those on a dose less than 600 mg and 6% in those taking over 600 mg. It has a very broad spectrum pharmacological activity blocking all types of dopamine receptors (D1 to D5), including D4, which is blocked little by other antipsychotics. Clozapine appears to exert its therapeutic effects by blocking a much lower proportion of D2 receptors (40 to 60%) than is the case with classical antipsychotics which occupy over 75%. EPS are more likely when 80% or more of the D2 receptors have been blocked.

Clozapine is particularly useful in treatment-resistant schizophrenia. About 60% of such patients benefit. Improvement can continue for up to one year. It has been associated with reduced suicide rate in schizophrenia when used long term and can lead to improvement in severe tardive dyskinesia. However, it can lead to troublesome side effects including sedation, excessive salivation, hypotension (fall in blood pressure), nausea, vomiting and fits. The usual dose range is 200 to 450 mg per day with a maximum of 900 mg per day.

Use of antipsychotic medication in people with learning disability

Traditional antipsychotics are not drugs of first choice due to their sedative effects, EPS, risk of tardive dyskinesia and worsening of seizure control. Neuroleptic malignant syndrome may be a particular risk in this group. National Institute for Clinical Excellence (NICE) guidance (NICE 2002) recommends that atypical antipsychotics should be considered as a first-line treatment of newly diagnosed schizophrenia and when discussion with the individual is not possible. The guidance also states that changing to an atypical antipsychotic is not necessary if a conventional antipsychotic controls symptoms adequately and there are no unacceptable side effects.

In those with learning disability, use of antipsychotic drugs is based mainly on observational studies or expert opinion and reports. Antipsychotics are used for treating psychotic conditions such as schizophrenia, paranoid states and mania where delusions, hallucinations, disturbed thinking and agitation may be prominent. Such drugs are also commonly used in a non-specific way for irritability, agitation, anxiety, aggression and self-injurious behaviour. Antipsychotics are also used for emergencies involving severe behavioural problems including physical aggression. Atypical antipsychotics such as risperidone, olanzapine, quetiapine and amisulpride have been used in those diagnosed as having pervasive developmental disorders (PDD) or autistic spectrum disorder mainly for behavioural management. For risperidone, for example, currently there has been only one randomised, controlled trial, that of McDougle et al. (1998). They performed a 12 week double-blind placebo controlled study in 31 adults with autistic disorder ($n = 17$) and pervasive developmental disorder not otherwise specified (PDD NOS) ($n = 14$). The mean dose range of risperidone was 1.5 to 4.5 mg per day. Side effects were mild with transient sedation in five patients. Other side effects included an increase in appetite, fatigue, dizziness and drooling. Risperidone was superior to placebo in reducing repetitive behaviour, aggression, anxiety/nervousness, depression, irritability and overall behavioural symptoms of autism. It is not possible to draw any robust conclusions regarding use of risperidone in patients with PDD based on this one study. Amisulpride and quetiapine have been anecdotally reported to be useful in autism.

Atypical antipsychotics, with their more favourable side-effect profile compared to traditional drugs such as haloperidol, may be useful in clinical practice for reducing the intensity and severity of behavioural symptoms such as aggression, irritability, nervousness and agitation. This would hopefully allow the person to participate more actively in social and learning activities as well as possibly allow behavioural approaches to be used more successfully. It is important that the initial dose of medication used in these circumstances is low and dose increments are gradual after careful assessment of benefits versus risks. It is particularly important to be vigilant for undue sedation during the day time as this could further impair thinking and learning and increase frustration leading to worsening of behaviour problems in some cases.

Guidance on antipsychotic drug reduction or withdrawal

Due to the lack of good research evidence for the effectiveness of antipsychotic medication in reducing maladaptive behaviour and concerns about side effects and use in people with learning disability who cannot give informed consent or report side effects, it is important to stop such medication when it is not beneficial. Although the dosage of antipsychotic medication can be successfully decreased or such medication stopped when it is not required, a minority suffer significant deterioration when dosages are decreased. Luchins et al. (1993) studied factors associated with reduction in antipsychotic medication dosage in adults with mental retardation residing in a 75-bed unit over a 5 year period. They found that the presence of a psychotic diagnosis was a significant variable in increased antipsychotic dosage. Use of alternative medication (carbamazepine, buspirone, lithium and propranolol) was helpful in allowing reduction of the dose of antipsychotic medication. The findings suggest that individuals with mental retardation who do not have psychoses are a suitable group for dose reduction and that the use of alternative medications facilitates this process.

Ahmed et al. (2000) conducted a randomised controlled trial to investigate factors influencing antipsychotic drug reduction in people with learning disabilities who had been prescribed such medication for behavioural reasons. Twelve of the 36 experimental subjects in this trial (33%) completed the full withdrawal programme of reducing the total dose by 25% every 4 weeks. A further seven (19%) were able to reduce the dose by at least 50%. The remaining 17 (48%) had to have their medication dose increased to baseline levels – ten after the initial 25% reduction, one after the 50% reduction and six after the 100% reduction. A limitation of this study was the small numbers involved in analysis. A double-blind study design was not used and the study was designed to reflect the factors that are important in real-life clinical situations when drug reduction is attempted. Drug reduction was associated with increased movement disorder consistent with the literature on tardive dyskinesia emerging on withdrawal of antipsychotic medication. Drug reduction was also associated with higher engagement in activity consistent with reduced sedative effects of medication. Interestingly drug reinstatement was not associated with deterioration of behaviour as rated from staff report or independent observations. Staff and environmental factors were important in distinguishing between the two groups. Drug reinstatement was associated with greater restriction and adaptation of the setting, less flexible staffing arrangements and less well developed policies and staff training for responding to difficult behaviour. Staff attitudes and apprehension were also important in determining drug reduction outcome. Thus the best predictors of failure were environmental, that is, lack of training, access to refresher courses, poor skill levels of staff and poor quality of the environment. In the group where medication was reinstated there were no major continuing behavioural problems, suggesting that in this group medication was possibly beneficial. In routine clinical practice dose reduction could be carried out more slowly than reported in the above study, especially when problematic environmental factors as described above are present.

Antidepressants

Depression is associated with a decrease in the level of serotonin and/or noradrenalin in the hippocampus and limbic regions of the brain. The precise cause of this decrease is unknown. Antidepressants work by increasing brain levels of serotonin and noradrenalin. This increase occurs within hours of taking an antidepressant, but there is a delay of at least 10 days for the improvement to be distinguishable from placebo and 4 to 6 weeks for full effect. The response rate to antidepressants alone is 60 to 70% and the placebo response rate is about 30%. The symptoms that respond best are low mood, loss of enjoyment, tiredness, poor appetite, sleep problems, guilt and pessimistic thoughts.

Guidelines for the use of antidepressants

The following guidelines illustrate current practice in the use of antidepressants for depression in the general population:

- *First episode*: a depressive episode may begin either suddenly or gradually. The duration of an untreated episode ranges from a few weeks to months or even years. It is important to continue medication at the same dose that was originally effective for at least six months *after* recovery (in practice a total of 9 months in all) to prevent the depression recurring.
- *Recurrent depression*: after one episode, 50 to 85% of patients will have another; after the second episode, 80 to 90% will have a third episode. About 20% develop a chronic form of depression. It is estimated that 10 to 15% of all patients hospitalised with depression eventually commit suicide. Factors that increase suicide risk include poor social support and isolation, older age, history of alcohol or substance abuse, history of prior suicide attempts and expressed suicidal intent with detailed plans of how to carry it out. Multiple episodes may require treatment for years. The chances of staying well are greatly increased by taking antidepressants. Antidepressants are effective, not addictive, are not known to lose their efficacy over time and are not known to cause new long-term side effects.

It is important not to stop antidepressants suddenly. They should be reduced slowly under supervision of a doctor to prevent unpleasant discontinuation effects. These include flu-like symptoms, 'shock-like' sensations, dizziness, insomnia, excessive (vivid) dreaming, irritability, crying spells, problems with concentration, memory and rarely movement disorders. Reducing the dose of antidepressant gradually over 4 to 6 weeks can prevent discontinuation reaction.

Types of antidepressants

Tricyclics or TCAs
Amitriptyline, imipramine and clomipramine are examples of tricyclics. Side effects include dry mouth, excessive sweating, constipation, sedation, blurring of vision, dizziness, postural hypotension, weight gain and urinary retention. They should be used with caution in those with glaucoma and prostate enlargement. Cardiac arrhythmias and heart block can occur and may be a factor in the sudden death of those with cardiac disease. These drugs may make

epilepsy worse. Due to the unfavourable side-effect profile, toxicity or lethality in overdose and the need to adjust the dose gradually by frequent monitoring, they are not generally used as first-line agents for the treatment of depression and anxiety disorders. Intolerable side effects can occur with low doses before beneficial effects, and thus patients may stop the drug too soon in the belief that it is not going to work. Tricyclic drugs have often been used in inadequate, low doses due to worsening of side effects on increasing the dose to a level where they are likely to have a beneficial effect on depression.

Selective serotonin re-uptake inhibitors (SSRIs)
Examples of SSRIs include fluoxetine (Prozac), paroxetine (Seroxat), citalopram (Cipramil), escitalopram (Cipralex) and sertraline (Lustral). Side effects are usually mild and transient and less severe than TCAs. They include headache, nausea, nervousness, diarrhoea, sleep difficulty and loss of appetite. SSRIs are also much safer than TCAs in cases of overdose. They are helpful in relieving anxiety symptoms within depression, panic disorder, obsessive–compulsive disorder, social phobia, post-traumatic stress disorder and bulimia nervosa. Fluoxetine has also been found useful for premenstrual dysphoric disorder or premenstrual tension.

Other types of antidepressants
- Serotonin noradrenalin re-uptake inhibitors (SNRIs), for example venlafaxine (Efexor).
- Noradrenergic and specific serotonergic antidepressants (NaSSAs), for example mirtazapine (Zispin).
- Selective noradrenaline re-uptake inhibitors (NARIs), for example reboxetine.
- Monoamine oxidase inhibitors (MAOIs), for example phenelzine (Nardil).
- Reversible monoamine oxidase inhibitors (RIMA), for example moclobemide.
- Other antidepressants include bupropion which has a similar side-effect profile as SSRIs but carries a risk of seizures, and trazodone.

Use of antidepressants in people with learning disability

There are many case reports of patients with learning disability and depression who have been treated successfully with SSRIs. Verhoeven et al. (2001), in an open trial with 20 subjects, showed that citalopram was effective in 60% of patients with learning disabilities (mental retardation) and depression. Treatment for one year on the effective dose prevented recurrence of depression. This study concluded that citalopram was a well-tolerated, safe and effective antidepressant in patients with learning disabilities suffering from depression. Clinical experience suggests that the use of such medication is safe due to their benign side-effect profile and ease of use. Additionally abnormal serotonin function has been thought to be associated with anxiety, impulsivity, aggression and goal-directed motivation. Serotonin may be involved in a variety of normal and abnormal behaviours such as stress responsiveness, impulsivity, anxiety, obsessive–compulsive symptoms and suicidal tendency associated with depression (Verhoeven and Tuinier 1999). Thus it has been suggested that some forms of behavioural problems such as stereotypies, self-injurious behaviour, aggressive behaviour and obsessive–compulsive symptoms may be responsive to treatment with serotonin-modulating compounds.

Hypnotics and anxiolytics

Benzodiazepines

Benzodiazepines, for example diazepam (valium), nitrazepam (mogadon), temazepam (normison) and lorazepam (ativan), are the most commonly used anxiolytics and hypnotics. Most anxiolytics (sedatives) will induce sleep when given at night and most hypnotics will sedate when given during the day. Dependence (both physical and psychological) and tolerance (needing a higher dose to obtain the same effect) occurs with these drugs. Thus treatment should be limited to the lowest possible dose for the shortest possible time.

The Committee of Safety of Medicines (CSM) advises that benzodiazepines should only be used for the short-term relief (2 to 4 weeks) of anxiety that is severely disabling or causing the individual unacceptable distress. Similarly they should only be used to treat insomnia or sleep disturbance that is severely disabling associated with extreme personal distress.

The main indications for these drugs are to induce sleep, reduce anxiety, control epilepsy, reduce withdrawal symptoms in alcohol dependency and as an adjunct in managing acutely disturbed behaviour. The most common side effects are drowsiness, lightheadedness, confusion, ataxia (unsteady gait), forgetfulness and dependence. A paradoxical increase in hostility and aggression can occur with effects ranging from talkativeness and excitement to aggressive and antisocial acts (British National Formulary 2004).

Withdrawal of benzodiazepines should be gradual. Abrupt withdrawal can lead to confusion, toxic psychosis, convulsions and delirium. Typical withdrawal symptoms may develop at any time, from a few hours up to 3 weeks after ceasing to take benzodiazepines, and consist of sleep disturbance, anxiety, loss of appetite, shakiness, excess sweating, tinnitus and perceptual disturbances.

Buspirone

Buspirone is a non-benzodiazepine anxiolytic. It acts by enhancing the action of serotonin at the 5-HT-1A receptor site. Its anti-anxiety effects develop within 1 to 2 weeks of treatment. The recommended dose is 5 to 10 mg three times daily. Tolerance and withdrawal symptoms do not develop. Buspirone does not relieve withdrawal symptoms due to benzodiazepines. Side effects include nausea, headaches and dizziness. Varying degrees of success with buspirone to combat aggression, self-injury and overarousal behaviour have been reported (Verhoeven and Tuinier 1996).

Beta blockers

Propranolol can be used for bodily symptoms of anxiety such as rapid heart beat (palpitations), shaking and sweating. The dose for anxiety is 40 mg once daily to 40 mg three times a day. Side effects include slowing of heart rate (bradycardia), heart failure, lowering of blood pressure, tiredness, insomnia with nightmares, coldness of the tips of fingers and toes, gastro-intestinal disturbances and worsening of psoriasis. It is contradicted in those with asthma, uncontrolled heart failure, marked bradycardia (low heart rate, i.e. below 55), low blood pressure and heart conduction defects or arrhythmias.

Sovner and Lowry (2001) highlighted the difficulties arising from lack of objective criteria to aid clinicians in deciding which specific psychotropic agents should be used in organic mental syndromes associated with learning disabilities. They proposed a category of 'overarousal' defined as 'a state of inappropriate alertness and readiness for action'. Overaroused individuals are in a state of hypervigilance with autonomic activation – a state of readiness for fight or flight. Beta blockers such as propranolol have been reported to be effective in modulating arousal. In the learning disabled population there is some evidence that beta blocker therapy can decrease self-injurious behaviour and aggression in autistic adults probably by decreasing arousal (Sovner and Lowry 2001).

Lithium

Lithium carbonate is a naturally occurring salt which has been found to have mood stabilising properties. It has been available since 1970. The most common indication for using lithium is in the prophylaxis of manic and depressive episodes, that is, in preventing recurrence of such episodes. It is also effective in reducing the frequency and severity of manic episodes. It has been shown to be effective in preventing recurrences of depression in patients with unipolar (recurrent) depression. Other uses include treatment of aggression in patients with dementia, learning disability and impulsive personality disorders (Andreasen and Black 2001).

Advantages
- Sixty to eighty percent response rate in acute mania
- Best studied mood stabiliser
- Appears to have a specific benefit in suicide prevention as has clozapine

Disadvantages
- Side effects may be intolerable for some
- Narrow therapeutic:toxic ratio resulting in severe toxic effects if blood levels become too high (over 1.5 mmol/l)

- Poor response in mixed states (that is, where both manic and depressive features are equally prominent) and rapid cycling bipolar illness, i.e. rapid mood swings with more than four episodes per year
- High relapse rates on abrupt discontinuation

Pre-lithium work-up
The following baseline investigations are recommended prior to commencing lithium: ECG, thyroid function tests, renal function tests (serum creatinine and urea), blood electrolytes and advice on reliable contraception in women of childbearing age if appropriate. Once stable it is important to check lithium levels every 3 to 6 months and thyroid function every 6 months. When stopping it is important to do this slowly over at least 1 month to prevent recurrence of the illness.

Short-term side effects
Side effects that occur in the short term include: mild gastrointestinal symptoms (discomfort in the stomach or loose motions, usually transient), thirst and polyuria (passing more urine), fine hand tremors, weight gain and oedema. Skin conditions such as psoriasis and acne may get worse.

Long-term side effects
Side effects that occur in the long term include underactive thyroid (clinical hypothyroidism occurs in 5 to 10% of patients). Those with pre-existing thyroid antibodies or a family history of thyroid disease are more at risk. Some patients report mental dulling or poor memory. Objective testing usually shows little change in memory with lithium use and in therapeutic doses lithium does not impair psychomotor coordination. Excessive thirst occurs in about 30% of patients. Chronic renal failure can occur rarely with long-term use.

Lithium toxicity
Diagnosis should be made based on clinical judgement and not just the blood levels of lithium. It is important to monitor blood levels regularly. Optimum levels are between 0.6 and 1.2 mmol/l. In prophylaxis the effective plasma level is lower (0.5 to 0.8 mmol/l). Toxic effects occur at levels above 1.5 mmol/l and include anorexia (loss of appetite), nausea, diarrhoea, vomiting, slurred speech, muscle weakness, drowsiness, ataxia ('drunken' gait), coarse tremor and muscle twitching.

Blood levels above 2 mmol/l result in increased disorientation, generalised muscle twitching, apathy, seizures and coma. Treatment here requires osmotic or forced alkaline diuresis. If the levels are above 3 mmol/l peritoneal or haemodialysis is often used to speed up the removal of lithium.

Use of lithium in people with learning disabilities
Sovner and Hurley (1981) reviewed the literature on the efficacy of lithium carbonate in the treatment of chronic behaviour disorders in adults with mental

retardation (learning disability). They concluded that there is some support for the use of lithium to manage behaviour disorders characterised by hyperactivity, aggression and/or self-mutilation. They recommend a drug-free trial once therapeutic effect has been achieved in order to assess the continued need for such treatment. Langee (1990) reported a 10 year retrospective study of 74 severely and profoundly mentally retarded institutionalised residents who had received lithium carbonate for various behaviour disorders. Thirty-one of the 74 patients with sustained reduction or elimination of behavioural symptoms were classified as lithium responders. Tyrer et al. (1984) reported a double-blind crossover trial lasting 5 months comparing the effects of lithium with placebo on aggressive behaviour. Twenty-five mentally handicapped (learning disabled) adults in hospital with persistent aggressive behaviour took part. All patients were receiving neuroleptic and/or anticonvulsant drugs which were continued during the trial. Seventeen of the patients showed greater improvement during the lithium phase compared to placebo. No patient became toxic during the investigation although lithium levels were maintained within the therapeutic range (0.5 to 0.8 mmol/l). This study suggests that lithium in combination with other medication is well tolerated and helpful in some people with learning disabilities and persistent aggression. Craft et al. (1987) in a double-blind trial compared the effect of lithium with placebo in 42 patients with learning disability. Seventy-three percent of patients showed a reduction in aggression during treatment lasting 4 months. There were no episodes of toxicity and no patients were withdrawn from the trial. They concluded that lithium was worth trying in patients presenting with repeated aggression where this had not been relieved by behavioural treatment or environmental measures such as more appropriate placement and increased occupation. Thus in the learning disabled population lithium may be beneficial in the treatment of long-standing aggression and hyperactivity in addition to its usual indications for use in bipolar affective disorder.

Mood stabilisers

Valproate

Valproate is available in two different formulations. Sodium valproate or Epilim is the preparation widely used for all forms of epilepsy as a first-line treatment. Valproate semi-sodium or Depakote is now increasingly used in the UK for mania, prophylaxis of bipolar disorder, mixed affective states and lithium non-responders. Valproate is thought to exert its effect by increasing the function of the inhibitory neurotransmitter gamma amino butyric acid (GABA).

Advantages of valproate semi-sodium
- Licensed for acute mania
- Efficacy across a spectrum of bipolar disorders, for example classic mania, mixed mania or rapid cycling bipolar disorder
- May be effective when lithium has failed

- Response is fast: within 1 to 4 days
- Efficacy is maintained over time
- Well tolerated

Disadvantages of valproate semi-sodium
- Further studies are needed to establish efficacy in prophylaxis

Side effects of valproate semi-sodium
It is generally well tolerated and most side effects are dose-related. Commonly reported side effects include gastrointestinal symptoms (for example nausea, poor appetite, vomiting, diarrhoea), weight gain, hair loss, fine postural tremor and sedation or drowsiness. Gastrointestinal side effects are less with the enteric-coated preparation of valproate. Less common side effects include rashes and haematological abnormalities with spontaneous bruising or bleeding. Rarely pancreatitis with acute abdominal pain has been reported. Liver dysfunction including fatal hepatic failure has also been described. This is a particular risk in children under 3 years of age and those with metabolic or degenerative disorders, organic brain disease or severe seizure disorders associated with mental retardation, usually in the first 6 months of therapy (British National Formulary 2004). Thus before treatment with valproate is initiated the patient should have a full blood count and liver function tests to measure liver enzymes. The latter should be measured frequently for the first 6 weeks and then at 6 monthly intervals thereafter. Neural tube defects have been reported with the use of valproate in the first trimester of pregnancy. Thus its use in pregnant women is not recommended. A fetal valproate syndrome has been described with cardiac and other congenital abnormalities and with jitteriness and seizures in the neonate (Cookson et al. 2002).

Carbamazepine

Carbamazepine is used in all forms of epilepsy except absence seizures. It is also used in mania, rapid cycling manic depressive illness and trigeminal neuralgia (pain). It may be more effective in rapid cycling bipolar disorder (four or more episodes per year) and those who respond poorly to lithium. It can be safely combined with antipsychotics especially when behavioural control is necessary (Andreasen and Black 2001). The exact mechanism of action is not known, but an antikindling effect resulting in reduced excitability of brain neurons is of interest.

Side effects
Reported side effects include nausea, vomiting, dizziness, drowsiness, headache, ataxia, confusion and agitation (in the elderly) and visual disturbances (especially double vision). A generalised rash can occur in 10 to 15% of patients, requiring a discontinuation of the medication. Reduced white blood cell counts

and other blood disorders including thrombocytopenia and aplastic anaemia can occur rarely. Carbamazepine should be avoided in the first trimester of pregnancy due to the possibility of neural tube defects in the fetus.

Many of these side effects can be avoided by starting with a low dose (100 to 200 mg, one to two times daily) and increasing it gradually. It is important to monitor full blood counts and electrolytes regularly. Clinical judgement is more important than blood levels in deciding on dose changes.

Use of mood stabilisers in people with learning disability

Valproate and carbamazepine may be useful in rapid cycling behavioural problems and outbursts of rage especially in those with electroencephalogram abnormalities. There is no direct relationship between blood levels and clinical response in mood disorders. Sovner (1989) reported five cases of bipolar disorder in adults with mental retardation (learning disability) treated with divalproex sodium. Two patients had chronic mania, two patients had rapid cycling illness (one of whom had an autistic disorder) and one patient had a classic bipolar disorder superimposed on an autistic disorder. Four of the patients showed a good response to valproate while the fifth patient had a moderate response.

Kastner et al. (1993) conducted an open trial of valproic acid in the treatment of affective symptoms in people with mental retardation (learning disability). Their criteria for treatment included the presence of three of the following four symptoms: irritability, sleep disturbance, aggressive or self-injurious behaviour and behavioural cycling. Eighteen patients completed the study. Fourteen patients (78%) responded favourably to treatment and were maintained on valproic acid for the 2 years of the study. A history of epilepsy or a suspicion of seizures was strongly associated with a favourable response to valproic acid. The results of this study suggest that people with mental retardation and concurrent affective disorders can be recognised by a cluster of developmentally appropriate atypical affective symptoms described above. In addition, such affective symptoms were successfully treated with valproate. This allowed discontinuation of neuroleptic medication in 90% of the patients who were on such medication in this study.

Reid et al. (1981) conducted a double-blind, placebo controlled, crossover trial of carbamazepine in 12 overactive adult patients with severe and profound mental retardation (learning disability). Patients who exhibited overactivity accompanied by some degree of mood elevation responded best. There was no relationship between response to carbamazepine and the presence or absence of epilepsy. This study suggests that there may be a small group of patients with severe learning disability and associated overactivity in whom carbamazepine might be clinically useful.

In conclusion valproate and carbamazepine may be particularly useful in the treatment of atypical or rapidly cycling bipolar disorders, which are more likely to be found in those with learning disability, especially in the severe and profound range. Sovner and Lowry (2001) proposed that individuals with chronic overactivity, boisterous or excited mood, sleep disturbance and distractibility may be suffering from chronic mania, a variant of an organic mood syndrome. They further speculate that antimanic anticonvulsants such as valproate and carbamazepine may be effective in this disorder.

Recent developments in the treatment of bipolar disorders include the use of newer anticonvulsants such as lamotrigine, topiramate and gabapentin and atypical antipsychotics particularly olanzapine, risperidone, clozapine and quetiapine. The latter are useful for the treatment of acute mania. Lamotrigine may be particularly useful in the treatment of bipolar depression and in some patients with rapid cycling bipolar disorder (Evins 2003).

Electroconvulsive therapy (ECT)

The National Institute for Clinical Excellence (NICE 2003) recommends that electroconvulsive therapy (ECT) should be used only to achieve rapid and short-term improvement of severe symptoms after an adequate trial of other treatment options has proven ineffective and/or when the condition is considered to be potentially life-threatening, in individuals with:

- Severe depressive illness, that is discrete episodes that are characterised by feelings of sadness, despair, loss of interest in daily life and discouragement. The severity of depressive illness is determined by the number, intensity and frequency or persistence of depressive symptoms and the presence of specific symptoms such as delusions, hallucinations and suicidal ideation.
- Catatonia, that is marked changes in muscle tone or activity that may alternate between the extremes of a deficit of movement (catatonic stupor) and excessive movement (catatonic excitement).
- A prolonged or severe manic episode characterised by elated, euphoric or irritable mood and increased energy.

Furthermore it is important that 'the decision as to whether ECT is clinically indicated is based on a documented assessment of the risks and potential benefits to the individual, including: the risks associated with the anaesthetic; current co morbidities; anticipated adverse events, particularly cognitive impairment; and the risks of not having treatment. Valid consent should be obtained in all cases where the individual has the ability to grant or refuse consent. In all situations where informed discussion and consent is not possible the individual's advocate and/or carer should be consulted'. ECT is usually given twice a week and a course usually involves between six and twelve treatments. Side effects immediately after treatment may include confusion, headache, nausea and muscle pain. The most troublesome long-term side effect is memory impairment. ECT may cause short- or long-term memory impairment for past events (retrograde amnesia) and current events (antero-grade amnesia). As this type of cognitive impairment is a feature of many mental health problems it may sometimes be difficult to differentiate the effects of ECT from those associated with the condition itself (NICE 2003).

ECT in people with learning disability

There are few reports on the use of ECT in patients with learning disability. Thuppal and Fink (1999) described the use of ECT in five patients with mental retardation and affective or psychotic disorders. ECT was successful in those who had previously responded poorly to drug therapy. There was no dispro-portionate increase in side effects due to learning disability. Van Waarde et al. (2001) conducted a literature review of the use of ECT in mental retardation (learning disability). They found 44 cases in the literature, most with diagnosed psychotic depression. In 84% of them, ECT was effective without excessive side effects. However, relapse occurred frequently (48%). In 16%, there were intolerable side effects and/or no improvement was seen. The reported case studies suggest that ECT may be of value in treating severe psychiatric disor-ders in people with learning disability and that the indications are similar to those in the general population. However, ethical and legal issues regarding the use of ECT in those who are unable to give informed consent probably unnecessarily limit its use in these patients. Further controlled trails are needed to firmly establish the efficacy and safety of ECT in those with learning disability.

Conclusion

Medication is an important form of intervention in the treatment of mental health disorders and associated behaviours. This chapter has provided insight into the classification of medication for people with learning disabilities and mental health disorders, the use of medication and its side effects. From a nursing perspective, it is important to observe safety in the administration of medication and to be able to identify the adverse effects of medication.

References

Ahmed, Z., Fraser, W., Kerr, M., et al. (2000) Reducing antipsychotic medication in people with learning disability. *British Journal of Psychiatry*, **174**, 42–46.

Andreasen, N. and Black, D. (2001) *Introductory Textbook of Psychiatry*, 3rd edition. Washington DC: American Psychiatric Press.

British National Formulary (2004) *British National Formulary*. London: British Medical Association and the Royal Pharmaceutical Society of Great Britain.

Brylewski, J. and Duggan, L. (1998) *Antipsychotic Medication for Challenging Behaviour in People with Learning Disability*. Oxford: The Cochrane Library.

Clarke, D., Kelley, S., Thinn, K. and Corbett, J. (1990) Psychotropic drugs and mental retardation. 1. Disabilities and the prescription of drugs for behaviour and for epilepsy in three residential settings. *Journal of Mental Deficiency Research*, **34**, 385–395.

Cookson, J., Taylor, D. and Katona, C. (2002) *Use of Drugs in Psychiatry*, 5th edition. London: Gaskell Press.

Craft, M., Ismail, I.A., Krishnamurti, D., et al. (1987) Lithium in the treatment of aggression in mentally handicapped patients. A double-blind trial. *British Journal of Psychiatry*, **150**, 685–689.

Deb, S. and Fraser, W. (1994) The use of psychotropic medication in people with learning disability. Towards rational prescribing. *Human Psychopharmacology*, **9**, 219–272.

Duggan, L. and Brylewski, J. (1999) Effectiveness of antipsychotic medication in people with intellectual disability and schizophrenia. A systematic review. *Journal of Intellectual Disability Research*, **43**, 94–105.

Evins, A.E. (2003) Efficacy of newer anticonvulsant medications in bipolar spectrum mood disorders. *Journal of Clinical Psychiatry*, **64**, 9–14.

Kastner, T., Finesmith, R. and Walsh, K. (1993) Long-term administration of valproic acid in the treatment of affective symptoms in people with mental retardation. *Journal of Clinical Psychopharmacology*, **13** (6), 448–451.

Langee, H.R. (1990) Retrospective study of lithium use for institutionalized mentally retarded individuals with behaviour disorders. *American Journal of Mental Retardation*, **94**, 448–452.

Luchins, D.J., Dojka, D.M. and Hanrahan, P. (1993) Factors associated with reduction in antipsychotic medication dosage in adults with mental retardation. *American Journal of Mental Retardation*, **98** (1), 165–172.

Matson, J.L., Bamburg, J.W., Mayville, E. and Logan, J.R. (2000) Tardive dyskinesia and developmental disabilities: an examination of demographics and topography in persons with dual diagnosis. *British Journal of Developmental Disabilities*, **46**, 119–130.

McDougle, C.J., Holmes, J.P., Carlson, D.C., Pelton, G.H., Cohen, D.J. and Price, L.H. (1998) A double-blind, placebo-controlled study of risperidone in adults with autistic disorder and other pervasive developmental disorders. *Archives of General Psychiatry*, **55** (7), 633–641.

Molyneaux, P., Emerson, E. and Caine, A. (2000) Prescription of psychotropic medication to people with intellectual disabilities in primary health care settings. *Journal of Applied Research in Intellectual Disability*, **12**, 46–57.

National Institute for Clinical Excellence (NICE) (2002) *Guidance on the Use of Newer (Atypical) Antipsychotic Drugs for the Treatment of Schizophrenia* www.nice.org.uk.

National Institute for Clinical Excellence (NICE) (2003) Guidance on the use of electroconvulsive therapy. Technology appraisal no. 50, April 2003. www.nice.org.uk.

Reid, A.H., Naylor, G.J. and Kay, D.S. (1981) A double-blind, placebo controlled, crossover trial of carbamazepine in overactive, severely mentally handicapped patients. *Psychological Medicine*, **11** (1), 109–113.

Reiss, S. and Aman, M. (1997) The international consensus process on psychopharmacology and intellectual disability. *Journal of Intellectual Disability Research*, **41**, 448–455.

Sovner, R. (1989) The use of valproate in the treatment of mentally retarded persons with typical and atypical bipolar disorders. *Journal of Clinical Psychiatry*, **50**, 40–43.

Sovner, R. and Hurley, A. (1981) The management of chronic behaviour disorders in mentally retarded adults with lithium carbonate. *Nervous and Mental Disease*, **169**, 191–195.

Sovner, R. and Lowry, M. (2001) Mood and affect as determinants of psychotropic drug therapy. In: A. Dosen and K. Day (Eds) *Treating Mental Illness and Behaviour Disorders in Children and Adults with Mental Retardation*. Washington DC: American Psychiatric Press.

Thompson, C. (1994) The use of high dose antipsychotic medication. Consensus statement. *British Journal of Psychiatry*, **164**, 448–458.

Thuppal, M. and Fink, M. (1999) Electroconvulsive therapy and mental retardation. *ECT*, **15** (2), 140–149.

Tyrer, S.P., Walsh, A., Edwards, D.E., Berney, T.P. and Stephens, D.A. (1984) Factors associated with a good response to lithium in aggressive mentally handicapped subjects. *Progress in Neuropsychopharmacological Biological Psychiatry*, **8**, 751–755.

van Waarde, J.A., Stolker, J.J. and van der Mast, R.C. (2001) ECT in mental retardation: a review. *Journal of ECT*, **17** (4), 236–243.

Verhoeven, W. and Tuinier, S. (1996) The effect of buspirone on challenging behaviour in mentally retarded patients: an open prospective multiple-case study. *Journal of Intellectual Disability Research*, **40**, 502–508.

Verhoeven, W. and Tuinier, S. (1999) Psychopharmacology of challenging behaviours. In: N. Bouras (Ed.) *Psychiatric and Behaviour Disorders in Developmental Disabilities and Mental Retardation*. Cambridge: Cambridge University Press.

Verhoeven, W.M., Veendrik-Meekes, M.J., Jacobs, G.A., van den Berg, Y.W. and Tuinier, S. (2001) Citalopram in mentally retarded patients with depression: a long-term clinical investigation. *European Psychiatry*, **16** (2), 104–108.

Further reading

Fraser, W. (1999) Psychopharmacology and people with learning disability. *Advances in Psychiatric Treatment*, **5**, 471–477.

Chapter 8

Psychosocial interventions

Psychosocial interventions form a major part of the therapy of people with dual diagnosis. This chapter will explore the use of traditional therapeutic frameworks, such as cognitive behaviour therapy, behaviour therapy and psychotherapy, and also some of the key emerging approaches, including their evidence bases. The need for developing clinical practice and practice-based evidence will also be highlighted.

Key themes

- Psychosocial interventions
- Evidence base for the intervention approaches
- Developing and improving clinical practice

Introduction

Helping people with learning disabilities who experience mental illness is an art and a science. It is an art because of the diverse roles that professionals and carers have to play in communicating and interacting with people with learning disabilities and the emphasis on the helper's perception of the person who may need help and the way the helper interacts with the person. Many experienced professionals are able to reflect on how they have been able to get through to a person with learning disabilities who required therapeutic help and tell success stories of the art of implementing interventions. Conversely, many professionals and carers recount how complex and difficult it is to implement and evaluate interventions and treatment approaches in this field. Helping people with dual diagnosis is also a science as the professional is expected to intervene using methods that can be evaluated. Nurses and other health and social care professionals are expected to have adequate understanding of the models of therapeutic interventions together with a relevant knowledge base, with appreciation of its effectiveness and the necessary skills and competence in its adaptation to people with learning disabilities. The following sections will explore the various psychosocial approaches that can help people with learning disabilities and mental illness.

Cognitive behaviour therapy

Cognitive behaviour therapy originates from the works of Albert Ellis (1962) who formulated Rational Emotive Therapy (RET) and Aaron Beck (1967) who studied the cognitive factors associated with depression. The last 40 years have seen a gradual development of cognitive therapeutic models of interventions, primarily in the field of mental health. In recent years there have been reports of its use in general medicine (in cancer and coronary heart problems) and also in treating psychosomatic illnesses.

According to Dobson and Dozois (2001) all cognitive behavioural therapies share three fundamental beliefs. The first is that *cognitive activity affects behaviour*. This is based on the belief that cognitive appraisals of events can affect the response to those events and that there is clinical value in modifying the content of these appraisals. The second is based on the belief that *cognitive activity may be monitored and altered*. It is assumed that the therapist is able to have access to cognitive activity and is fully able to map these activities, which can be altered. The third is that the *desired behaviour change may be affected through cognitive change*. It is assumed that the behaviour change may be the result of overt reinforcement contingencies that can alter the behaviour and also the mediational influences on cognitive restructuring and behaviour change.

The term *cognitive behaviour therapy* (CBT) is used to describe a range of therapeutic models that share the same aims and characteristics. The key underlying assumptions of cognitive behaviour approaches focus on the following:

- Thoughts, images, perceptions and other cognitive mediating events affect overt behaviour as well as emotions.
- These mediating conditions occur in a systematic, structured manner to facilitate the change in behaviour and emotions.
- People are active learners, not just passive recipients of environmental influence. To some extent they create their own learning environment and sometimes their specific learning histories result in cognitive dysfunction.
- Treatment goals centre around creating new adaptive learning opportunities to overcome cognitive dysfunctions and to produce positive changes for the person, which can be generalised and maintained outside the clinical setting.
- The person has an understanding of the intervention strategies and goals, and participates in planning and defining these.

(Stenfert Kroese 1997)

Literature concerning the use of CBT in people with learning disabilities is scarce at present. Lindsay et al. (1997) highlight the key reasons for the lack of adequate research in the application of CBT in people with learning disabilities. They consist of: (1) the notion that people with learning disabilities are a devalued population and are of little interest to the research community; (2) the assumption that people with learning disabilities do not have as stable and potent cognitions as those without learning disabilities and therefore it will be difficult to conclude that changes are as a result of clinical manipulations; (3) the notion that the manifestation of mental illness in people with learning disabilities is the same as in those without any learning disabilities and this may have barred the need for any focused research in this population. In addition to these, the inability of the person with a learning disability to self-report may have led to the lack of adequate research using CBT models. However, in recent years professionals are using CBT models in practice with people with learning disabilities and these are laying the foundations of an evidence base (however limited). Some of the important research findings in the use of a range of CBTs are being explored in relation to the treatment of various mental health disorders.

The evidence base regarding the application of CBT for treating anxiety related illnesses in people with learning disability is limited. Lindsay et al. (1997) propose an adapted model for treating anxiety disorders based on CBT involving a number of steps:

(1) Setting an agenda: discussion with the client concerning the possible steps of the treatment in simple language and possibly with visual cues. Lindsay et al. suggest that doing this may allow clients to understand the various concepts involved and may also allow them to organise the difficult materials in a systematic and simple way.
(2) Isolating negative thoughts: this can be a difficult phase for clients. Some people may be able to report negative thoughts through therapeutic interviews. Role-play sessions can also help the client to bring out the anxiety provoking negative thoughts and feelings. Lindsay et al. suggest an interesting method of role reversal of the client and therapist. In this context, the client as therapist can ask what 'the client' is thinking, and the 'therapist' could then ask leading questions of 'the client'. Lindsay et al. state that this method may be useful in revealing a clear picture of the nature of thoughts that may be important to the client.
(3) Eliciting underlying symptoms: by identifying the themes across automatic thoughts, such as identifying the symptoms of sleeplessness, fear, panic attacks and other behavioural symptoms.
(4) Testing the accuracy of cognitions: by using simple and direct methods of verifying the accuracy of the cognitions. This may be done by verbally reflecting the thoughts back to the client in a simple form using humour and stories to check accuracy.
(5) Generating alternative cognitions: by using the converse of negative thoughts. For example, if the client says, 'People are laughing at me when standing at a bus stop', the converse of the thought here will be 'No one is looking at me, no one is bothered about me'.

(6) Monitoring thoughts and feelings: this involves the use of simple tools such as cartoon representations of the emotion (such as happy, embarrassed, sad) to monitor thoughts and feelings.

(7) Role-play: anxiety provoking situations can be re-enacted using role play, to help clients understand the relationship between their thoughts and anxiety-related feelings and behaviours.

(8) Homework: setting homework is an important task. Lindsay et al. argue that this will help to monitor the extent of maladaptive thinking that has occurred during the week and provide situations in which more adaptive responses can be practised.

Several reports have appeared on the assessment of depression in this client group and there is a pressing need for more research into treatment of depression in people with learning disability. The two case studies by Lindsay et al. (1993) of individuals with mild intellectual disability illustrate the clinical applications. All the elements of CBT for depression were maintained and simplified. Both subjects were able to monitor their feelings of depression and the frequency of suicidal thoughts was monitored. Individuals saw improvements in both cases on the Zung depression inventory and on the daily monitoring of depressive feelings. This is an encouraging approach to the treatment of depression in this client group and demands further exploration through larger-scale controlled studies.

Dagnan and Chadwick (1997) discuss the Antecedent–Belief–Consequence model as a simple cognitive intervention strategy that can have an effective role in the treatment of mood disorders. The key stages of this model consist of (1) the antecedent phase, which focuses on an event, the client's attention to this event and the description of this event; (2) the belief phase, which focuses on the interpretation, appraisal or evaluation of the event; and (3) the consequence phase, which focuses on the emotional or the behavioural responses of the client.

In recent years CBTs have been applied to psychotic symptoms, with some reports of positive results. There is little in the literature to suggest that such techniques have been used to help people with learning disabilities that experience psychosis. Legget et al. (1997), however, attempted to explore whether teaching psychological strategies for managing auditory hallucinations in people with learning disabilities is effective. A case report describes the use of a cognitive behavioural strategy with a woman with mild learning disabilities. A number of benefits of the intervention are noted including decreases in subjective distress and use of pro re nata (PRN) (when required) medication, as well as improved mood and reported increases in the use of positive coping strategies and self-esteem.

Anger management

The manifestation of mental health disorder in people with learning disabilities may take the form of severe aggressive behaviour consisting of physical

Box 8.1   Anger management course content (adapted from Moore et al. 1997).

- Session 1: Introductions
  Familiarisation of group, learning names, setting group rules, for example confidentiality.
- Session 2: Starting to talk about feelings
  Looking together in small groups at pictures of people displaying different emotions. Groups to identify emotions and to talk about the experience of these emotions.
- Sessions 3: More about feelings
  The 'I feel . . .' game; someone reads a statement about an event and each person in the small group talks about how the situation described might have made him or her feel. In the large group, start to make connections between feelings and actions.
- Session 4: Think about anger
  What makes people angry? Demonstrate role plays with the facilitators. Learn about the signs of anger in other people. Take individual Polaroid photographs of each other smiling and looking angry.
- Session 5: What do we do with angry feelings?
  Explore the functions of anger and how it is expressed. What can we do if other people are getting angry? Use role plays by facilitators with audience participation; group members join in with suggestions of what might make the situation better.
- Session 6: Recognising own anger and that in others
  Practise using the most popular techniques from week 5 role plays between group members. Find out what works best for each person.
- Session 7: Practising anger management
  Make a video of how we deal with anger; everyone else has a chance to manage a situation where someone else is angry and to demonstrate a way of expressing their feelings.
- Session 8: Practising anger management
  More practice.
- Session 9: Review of achievements
  Share what has been learned. Talk about how people felt about the course.

aggression toward others, destruction of property and verbal aggression. The work of Raymond Novaco (1975) offered the first use of CBT in anger management and this has been modified over the years. The aim of anger management training is to develop coping skills so that the individual is able to appraise the anger provoking situations, cognitively process this information and respond with socially appropriate and adaptive behaviour. The key components of anger management training consist of (1) cognitive restructuring, (2) arousal reduction and (3) behavioural skills training (Black et al. 1997).

Psychologists and some behaviour specialist nurses organise anger management groups or individual sessions for people with dual diagnosis and severe aggressive behaviour. Moore et al. (1997) describe the process of conducting an anger management group with people with learning disabilities; a 9 week course consisting of nine sessions with a set pattern is indicated in Box 8.1.

Whilst conducting an anger management group for people with learning disabilities, it is important that care staff are able to attend all the sessions. Participation in anger management groups will allow a person with learning disability to:

- Gain positive experiences, from participation in a group
- Develop an understanding of what anger is and how it affects us all
- Learn some tricks to help deal with feeling angry so that situations are not made worse by the way anger is expressed
- Feel like an 'expert' instead of feeling out of control

It is important that nurses or key support workers attend the anger management group along with the person with learning disability. This will allow the person to:

- Learn from participation in the group experience
- Develop an understanding of what makes clients angry from the client's perspective
- Learn from clients what helps and what does not help when they are angry

The evidence base for anger management and its effectiveness in people with learning disabilities is growing. A component analysis (Benson 1986) of a cognitive behavioural anger management programme was conducted with adults with learning disabilities attending vocational training programmes. Self-control training was given in one of four groups: relaxation training, self-instruction, problem solving and a combined anger management condition. The dependent measures included self-reports, ratings of video-taped role plays and supervisor ratings. The results revealed decreases in aggressive responding over time and no significant differences between groups. The study suggests that anger management training with mentally retarded adults may be effective.

Rose et al. (2000) describe an evaluation of group intervention for reducing inappropriately expressed anger (in the form of aggression) in people with intellectual disabilities. Group intervention was compared with a non-treatment group consisting of people referred to the group but who had to wait to participate. Participants were accompanied by a support worker and more collaborative procedures were devised. A reduction in expressed anger and measured levels of depression occurred after group treatment. Reductions in expressed anger were maintained at 6 and 12 months follow up. However, scores on the depression scale tended to increase on follow up. While caution must be expressed when considering these results, group therapy shows promise for reducing inappropriately expressed anger in people with intellectual disabilities.

Lindsay et al. (1998) undertook a study of three individuals with learning disabilities who were exhibiting aggressive behaviour. The exploration of attitudes to anger and aggression included direct observation, self-recording of frequency of aggressive incidents, self-recording of feelings of aggression provocation, role plays and provocation inventories. Treatment approaches included two forms of relaxation [Brief Relaxation Therapy (BRT) and Abbreviated Progressive Relaxation (APR)], discussions and exercises on the understanding of emotion and role plays. The findings raise possibilities for the potential to tailor intervention programmes to individual needs by undertaking an initial comprehensive assessment of individuals' difficulties.

Willner et al. (2002) undertook a randomised controlled trial of the efficacy of a cognitive behavioural anger management group for clients with learning disabilities. Fourteen clients with learning disabilities referred for anger management were randomly assigned to a treatment and a waiting list group. Treatment consisted of nine 2 hour group sessions, using brainstorming, role play and homework. Topics addressed included the triggers that evoke anger, physiological and behavioural components of anger, cognitive and behavioural strategies to avoid the build up of anger and for coping with anger provoking situations and acceptable ways of displaying anger. The intervention was evaluated using two inventories of anger provoking situations, and was completed independently by both clients and careers. Clients in the treatment group improved on both client and carer ratings, relative to their own pre-treatment scores and to the control group post treatment. The degree of improvement within treatment was strongly correlated with verbal IQ. Clients in the treatment group showed further improvement relative to their own pre-treatment scores at 3 months follow up.

CBT approaches can be useful in working with people with dual diagnosis. There is a need for research studies looking at the utilisation and effectiveness of the various cognitive therapeutic models. Health and social care professionals need to document single case studies and group studies in order to develop the model of practice-based evidence.

Behaviour therapy

Behaviour therapy is based on the behavioural school of thought in psychology based on the works of Pavlov, Watson and Skinner, and others. Behaviour therapy has in some ways dominated the treatment realm in the field of learning disabilities because of its objective principles and methods and through its commanding role in teaching and maintaining adaptive behavioural skills.

The key principle of behaviour therapy is based on the assumption that behaviour is primarily affected by conditions existing in the person's environment, rather than the psychic/mind dynamics. It is believed that behaviour is a spontaneous response in relation to environmental stimuli and a person learns to use these behavioural responses through reinforcement, which increases the probability of the response occuring repeatedly.

The intervention strategies using behaviour therapy principles consist of key stages:

- Objective/operational definition of the target behaviour (to be increased or decreased).

- Assessment of the target behaviour using the Antecedent–Behaviour–Consequence framework (A–B–C) to identify the pattern, frequency and duration of the behaviour.
- Functional analysis of behaviour, which would help to formulate hypotheses of the causative factors of the target behaviour and to systematically approach this through the use of a range of skills teaching and/or techniques of reinforcement schedules.
- Intervention plans consist of detailed goals and strategies, which are constantly evaluated against baseline measures of the target behaviour.

Over the years behaviour therapy has undergone modifications and current principles of applied behaviour analysis tend to address the issues of intervention from a bi-psychosocial perspective, emphasising the rationale for the objectivity of behaviour as well as identification of the causative factors of or trigger factors for inappropriate behaviours or emotional problems. Behaviour therapy has moved away from the elimination or suppression of inappropriate behaviours to focus on teaching adaptive skills and social behaviours, thus promoting physical, psychological and social well-being.

Systematic desensitisation

Developed by Joseph Wolpe (1958) systematic desensitisation (SD) is a useful therapy for treating anxiety. This is a behavioural treatment procedure where a client is gradually exposed (through imagination or in real life) to a hierarchy of anxiety provoking stimuli. This is done in the context of maintaining a state of calm through deep muscle relaxation or by other relaxation procedures. The advantage of SD is that it can be used for people with learning disabilities who may have limited imaginary skills, exposing them to anxiety provoking stimuli in vivo (in real life contexts). Pleasurable activities such as eating or drinking or being with a favourite person can be used instead of the relaxation procedure to enable the person to remain in a state of calm whilst being exposed to the anxiety provoking stimuli. Individuals can also carry out SD by themselves, which is known as systematic self-desensitisation where the person progresses through the various desensitisation stages. This form of SD can be used to treat problematic fears such as fear of flying.

A modified approach has been used to treat individuals who suffer anxiety, specifically fear of dogs. Dixon and Gunary (1986) recruited to a group treatment programme 12 adults living in a mental handicap hospital for whom fear of dogs was a problem. Treatment involved gradual desensitisation over a period of 21 weekly sessions, making use of modelling procedures and exposure to four different dogs. At the end of the treatment all members showed some improvement in coping with their anxiety in the presence of dogs. This improvement was maintained after 9 months in those who had an opportunity to experience dogs regularly. The study fails to report how many of the recruited sample completed treatment and also there are insufficient details about the level of the anxiety or fear experienced by the individuals when they were recruited to the study.

Lindsay et al. (1988) described the development of a group anxiety management treatment incorporating training and exposure treatments for dog phobia with people with intellectual disabilities. The treatment procedures had several components including increased contact with dogs; changing dogs as treatment progresses; graded exposure to dogs, eliciting anxiety from an early stage in the programme; modelling reasonable reactions to dogs; encouraging individuals to have control over dogs; and promoting generalisation of coping behaviours. The procedures are illustrated by the cases of two women who were assessed on overall ratings of fear, number of positive approaches to a dog, number of negative reactions to a dog and self-assessments of anxiety. Both women responded to treatment. The results are discussed in terms of the patterning of the women's responses as treatment progressed. The study suggests that the exposure treatments may be a successful means of helping people with intellectual disabilities overcome their phobic anxiety.

Relaxation training

Relaxation training is used for anxiety management and its methods range from progressive muscle relaxation, where several muscle groups are individually tensed and relaxed, to imagery-based procedures, yoga and meditation. Benson and Havercamp (1999) suggest that relaxation training can be a primary intervention technique for managing generalised anxiety or it can be part of a treatment package. Relaxation techniques such as progressive relaxation developed by Jacobson (1929) and abbreviated progressive relaxation (Bernstein and Borkovec 1973) have been used with people with learning disabilities. Studies by Lindsay et al. (1989) comparing different anxiety treatments for adults with moderate and severe learning disabilities, Lindsay and Baty (1986) looking at group relaxation training and Calamari et al. (1987) evaluating multiple component relaxation training all suggest the use of relaxation techniques for people with learning disabilities. The following case example of Nathan highlights the role of relaxation in anxiety management.

Nathan is a 32-year-old man with mild learning disabilities (estimated full scale IQ 68). He was referred to the local health care services with a 2 year history of increased stress involving disturbed sleep, increased irritability and increasing insecurity and worry concerning routine daily activities that did not worry him before. He became quite particular about knowing which staff member was on the rota each day and felt anxious and panicky when alone. He lived in a bed-sit apartment with minimum support from a community team for adults with learning disabilities, and with only limited help at night consisting mainly of telephone support. Due to his increasing anxiety, Nathan avoided going out on his own and thus was increasingly isolating himself. He described panic attacks when he felt panicky, shaky, sweaty and dizzy together with thoughts that he might 'pass out' due to his rapid heart beat (palpitations) and rapid breathing when panicky. Such attacks occurred both at home when he was on his own and when he went to noisy crowded places such as supermarkets and local pubs. Prior to the onset of the anxiety, Nathan had been doing a lot of work at college and actively participating in a local advocacy group for people with learning disabilities. He was 'on the go' all the time and found it difficult to relax. Due to his good adaptive and independent living skills, his support team had been giving him much more choice about what he wanted to do on a day-to-day basis. Nathan had started a friendship with a young woman who also had mild learning disabilities. He found that his girlfriend had become demanding and jealous if he talked to any other young women. He had limited knowledge of sexuality and had had no previous sexual experience. Nathan had always been a worrier but had projected a confident outward 'front'. It became apparent that due to his outward confidence he was expected to be decisive and help sort out other peers' problems. He had always found it difficult to say 'no' to any requests for help and tried hard to please others. Thus he would often go along with other people's wishes rather than be appropriately assertive in a calm way and confidently state his point of view.

Interventions for Nathan involved:

- Education about anxiety; panic attacks and avoidance which are behavioural responses to the anxiety; education about healthy sexual relationships and sex education.
- Learning anxiety management and relaxation techniques.
- Graded exposure to situations that he was beginning to avoid.
- Assertiveness training and anger management techniques; joining a local time-limited anxiety management group where he met peers with similar difficulties and learnt to share his worries and realise that he was not the only one with an anxiety problem.
- Learning to recognise his strengths, 'pat himself on the back' for his achievements and improve his self-esteem and self-confidence.

Lindsay et al. (1989) explored anxiety treatments for adults who have moderate and severe learning disability by undertaking a study based on the simplification of a technique called progressive relaxation. They identified the problems of previous studies in which anxiety is measured indirectly, for example through a decrease in hyperactivity, and attempted to overcome this by using direct measures of anxiety and relaxation before treatment, during treatment and after treatment had finished. Fifty people with moderate and severe learning disability (IQ 30 to 55) were randomly allocated to five groups: individual behavioural relaxation training, individual abbreviated progressive relaxation training, group behavioural relaxation training, group abbreviated progressive relaxation and a control group. Anxiety was measured in accordance with the behavioural anxiety scale. Treatment lasted for 12 sessions for all groups; for subjects seen individually each session lasted between 30 and 45 minutes and for those seen in groups between 60 and 95 minutes. The study demonstrated that group behavioural relaxation training is an effective anxiety treatment in the short term. This study used a sound methodological approach to explore the different methods of anxiety management. It would be of further interest to see whether this intervention proves useful for managing anxiety in the longer term and whether regular sessions would be required to sustain the improvement.

In a study consisting of three case reports, Lindsay and Baty (1986) described the application of behavioural relaxation training as an intervention for anxiety in individuals with learning difficulties. The intervention involved training in and imitation of a series of relaxed behaviours. The participants were assessed on behavioural ratings and on a physiological rating (pulse rate) before and after treatment. The authors report that the participants all reacted positively in terms of increased relaxation and reduction in anxiety post treatment and highlight the potential usefulness of this approach among individuals with learning disabilities due to the simple nature of the participation required by the client.

Modelling

Modelling or observational learning involves an individual observing a peer who is performing the behaviour appropriately. Modelling is widely used in our daily interactions and behaviours, and parents use modelling to teach language and skills to their children. It is a useful technique in teaching people to manage problems such as stress, anxiety and fear. It can be used with people with learning disabilities in one-to-one interactions or in a group context. What is essential in modelling is for the person to observe a peer showing acceptable or culturally appropriate behaviours in dealing with a situation or as a response to stress or anxiety. A systematic procedure should be followed in the use of modelling, i.e. the setting, individual or group sessions, types of acceptable behaviours to be observed and the necessary instructions and guidance to be provided should be predetermined prior to a session. Modelling can also be introduced through films and video clips, which is known as symbolic modelling.

Social skills training

Socialisation and social skills are important aspects of an individual's development and behaviour. The evidence base stressing the relationship between social skills and psychopathology in people with learning disability is gradually emerging. For example, Helsel and Matson (1988) suggest that social skills training is important as part of an overall package in the treatment of depression. Laman and Reiss (1987) also identify the need for providing social support and encouraging social skills in dealing with low mood. Matson et al. (1998) stress the link between lack of social skills and psychopathology in people with severe and profound learning disabilities and emphasise the need for teaching positive behaviour and skills. We know that mental health is not just the absence of illness symptoms but also the capacity and capability of the person to deal with the stress and strain of living in a social world. Many people with learning disabilities have limited opportunities for developing social networks, socialisation, and the development of social behaviour and related skills, which is a key stress factor in the cause of mood disorders such as depression.

Social skills training will provide people with learning difficulties with new skills and encourage positive behaviour in dealing with social interactions and help in the everyday socialisation process and the development of a social network.

Counselling

The term counselling is broadly used and defined, and arriving at a concise definition can be difficult. Counselling is a way of helping others adjust to problems that distress them or make them unhappy and empowering them to make appropriate decisions in the face of life's problems. Different forms of counselling emphasise the individual's resources or strengths rather than psychopathology, with a focus on a reflective, experiential process. Here the patient's concerns are rephrased and clarified in order that he or she may develop a greater sense of well-being and cope with life's difficulties differently. There is emphasis on mental health promotion rather than 'treating disorders' (Department of Health 2001).

Psychodynamic approaches

Psychodynamic approaches focus on psychoanalysis. Psychotherapy is based on psychoanalytic approaches as proposed by Sigmund Freud. Psychotherapy has been in use for over a hundred years, but it still remains a complex therapeutic procedure based on the skill of the therapist conducting it. Various definitions have been proposed for psychotherapy, and some of the important ones are considered here in order to shed light on it. Strupp (1978) describes psychotherapy as an interpersonal process designed to bring about modifications of feelings, cognitions, attitudes and behaviour that have proven troublesome to the person seeking help from a trained professional. Storr (1979) defines psychotherapy as the art of alleviating personal difficulties through the agency of words and a personal, professional relationship.

Both definitions focus on the interaction and relationship with the therapist and the nature of the therapist as a trained professional in the use of psychotherapy. As psychodynamic approaches focus on the expression of thoughts and feelings using verbal language, its application to people with learning disabilities is a professionally challenging option. The works of Valerie Sinason (1992), Waitman and Conboy-Hill (1992), De Groef and Heinemann (1999) and Sheila Hollins (2001) provide an insight into the application of psychotherapy to people with learning disabilities.

Rather than concentrating primarily on symptoms and changing the symptoms, psychodynamic approaches focus on bringing about more radical changes in the personality or resolution of unconscious conflicts. The relationship between the patient and the therapist is an important part of therapy and this is seen as a vehicle for change in the patient. According to psychodynamic approaches, depression stems from the relationship with parents or early childhood experiences. It is suggested that an 'injury' may be caused by the relationship with the mother due to separation, loss, abandonment or lack of emotional responses from the mother. The child may learn to internalise and be dependent on the mother figure, and as the child grows up he or she becomes overly dependent on significant other people such as paid carers.

The discussion in this section is also about psychodynamic principles and their possible applications in the field of learning disabilities. Traditionally the ideal psychotherapy candidate was thought to be young, intelligent and articulate – not a description that fits a person with learning disability (Hollins 2003). *Psychoanalytic psychotherapy* is a longer-term therapy (usually a year or more) with the aim of allowing unconscious conflicts to be re-enacted in the relationship between the therapist and the client. In attempting to understand and look below the surface of the presenting complaints, the therapist generally offers test interpretations. The conflicts are 'worked through' within the therapeutic relationship. Psychodynamic therapy makes use of transference and countertransference of feelings in the relationship between therapist and client. Brown and Pedder (1991) in their book *Introduction to Psychotherapy* state that there are three key elements in the therapist–client relationship. These are the therapeutic or working alliance, transference and countertransference. The therapeutic or working alliance involves establishing a good rapport and a safe, secure and trusting relationship. This is fostered by friendliness, courtesy, reliability and being non-judgemental. The so-called non-specific factors in therapy, that is accurate empathy, warmth, genuineness, respect and unconditional positive regard, are particularly important here. The term transference refers to the tendency to respond to new relationships according to patterns or templates derived from important key past relationships, for example with parents.

A person who has been brought up by a strict parent might expect other adults or people in authority to behave in the same way towards them. Thus one transfers feelings and attitudes developed in previous similar experiences to the present relationship with a different person. Within psychotherapy the client may experience feelings towards the therapist as if he/she were an important figure from the client's past. Thus transference becomes a tool for investigating the forgotten and repressed past (Brown and Pedder 1991). Countertransference refers to the therapist's feelings and attitudes towards the client. These may be a reflection of what the client is experiencing and can thus be helpful in deepening the emotional understanding of the client. On the other hand such feelings may be due to the client reminding the therapist of important figures in the therapist's past. Thus the therapist may feel unduly angry towards the client for reasons that have little to do with the interaction with the client in the 'here and now'. If the therapist is unaware of where these feelings are coming from, he or she may react in a way that is unhelpful to the client. Brown and Pedder (1991) comment that it is assumed that a degree of introspection, average intelligence and verbal fluency are desirable for such therapy. Otherwise clients would find it difficult to reflect on their feelings and communicate this verbally with the potential for enacting them behaviourally, that is 'acting out'.

Hollins (2003) comments that a common assumption in the field of learning disabilities is that the intellectual impairment of the person will prevent him or her from attaining 'meaningful, emotional engagement'. She further states that part of the assessment interview for dynamic psychotherapy should include an honest appraisal by the therapist of his or her own feelings and reactions to the person with learning disabilities. The difficulty of establishing a therapeutic dialogue in the presence of communication difficulties has been seen as a barrier to people with learning disabilities having access to, or making effective use of, psychotherapy. However, art therapists and related disciplines have a long history of working through other means of expression than speech (Royal College of Psychiatrists 2004).

Psychological therapy services are a vital component of a comprehensive mental health service. There is, however, no formal training for learning disability psychotherapists and little specific psychotherapy service provision within learning disability mental health services (Royal College of Psychiatrists 2004). Professions such as nursing and social work which are in a good position to develop some basic psychotherapeutic interventions for people with learning disabilities are presently not equipped to do so by their basic training and the lack of a strategy or career pathway in post-qualification training.

People in distress generally have the option of using their own personal resources to cope or turn to others for support, advice and other forms of help, traditionally family, friends, community members, doctors or priests. A person with learning disability may have limited personal resources to cope with ordinary life stresses and may not have the ability to ask others for help due to limited communication or lack of adequate good quality support from others. Traditional treatments for psychological problems in people with learning disabilities have tended towards behavioural management, skills training and medication. Over the past 15 years, there has been a small but growing interest in extending the application of psychotherapeutic interventions to include people with learning disabilities. Psychotherapy has been demonstrated to be an effective form of treatment for people with psychological problems. However, there is considerable resistance to attempts to generalise these findings to people with intellectual disabilities.

Publication of several case studies in the late 1980s and early 1990s has provided some evidence for the benefit of various psychotherapeutic approaches in people with learning disabilities. However, there are only few outcome studies. Frankish (1992) reports the findings of psychodynamic therapy with a 6-year-old child with learning disabilities with behaviour problems in a one-to-one therapeutic setting. Beail and Warden (1996) present some preliminary data on nine men and one woman (18 to 49 years age range). The reasons for referral were aggressive behaviour (four people), sexually inappropriate behaviour (three people) and psychotic or bizarre behaviour (three people). This study also used specific outcome measures and reported significant reductions in psychological symptoms and an increase in self-esteem. Beail (1998) reports on the outcome of individual psychoanalytical therapy provided in normal clinical practice for 25 men with intellectual disabilities who were referred for behaviour problems. Of the 25 participants in the study, 20 completed treatment. In almost all cases the problem behaviour was eliminated and this was maintained at 6 months follow up.

Berry (2003) describes four cases of long-term treatment using psychodynamic therapy for challenging behaviour in a large institution for people with learning disabilities in Germany. A meta analysis of studies relating to psychotherapy of people with learning disabilities conducted by Prout and Nowak-Drabik (2003) reports a wide range of designs, types of interventions and participants involved. The overall analysis indicates that psychotherapy of people with learning disabilities produced a moderate amount of change and is moderately effective or beneficial.

Due to the emphasis of using spoken language as a medium of interaction in psychotherapy, its application to people with learning disabilities was ignored for many years. The recent report from the Royal College of Psychiatrists on *Psychotherapy and Learning Disability* (2004) provided the much needed background and emphasis on the use of psychotherapy of people with learning disabilities. This report suggests the need for psychotherapy to focus not only on mental health and emotional difficulties but also on issues of impairment, disability and handicap. It comments that current service provision of psychotherapy services for clients with learning disabilities in the UK ranges from highly specialised services, providing individual and group psychoanalytic therapy, to individuals or groups of clinicians who facilitate psychotherapeutic understanding in the day-to-day work of carers, professionals and support staff. The report further states that 'some of the more specialist expertise needed for effective psychotherapy for people with learning disabilities will be in establishing a productive treatment alliance through the development of an effective "language" and therapeutic context'. The process of assessment may be more prolonged and will involve more people than in generic services. Specific issues may require more attention, such as consent or the practicalities of therapy. Adaptation and flexibility of therapeutic approach are essential; this may often stretch or conflict with some of the common and traditional tenets of psychotherapy. The importance of working with the whole system around an individual is highlighted. The application of psychotherapy to people with learning disabilities requires modifications, and the evidence base needs to emerge with practice examples and research studies looking at the process and outcomes of therapy.

Solution-focused brief therapy (SFBT)

Solution-focused brief therapy (SFBT) is a psychotherapeutic approach based on:

- Finding out what clients want to change and
- Discovering resources already existing within clients which can be used to help them make the changes they want (de Shazer et al. 1986)

It is an approach of 'solution building' rather than 'problem solving' (Iveson 2002) and requires that therapists work hard not to impose their own theory of how best to achieve the changes the client wants. The therapist adopts a 'one-down' position and maximises the client's role as expert in his/her own life. Bliss (2002) argues that SFBT puts the person with learning disabilities at the centre of therapeutic interaction by listening very closely to the individual's view of what things would be like if the problems were no longer influential in his or her life.

SFBT pays attention to the following information:

(1) Pre-session change: have any positive changes occurred between receiving the letter of appointment and attending the appointment? It is important that these changes are noticed because they can be attributed directly to clients helping themselves, and can form important building blocks to future solutions.

(2) Non-problem talk: in keeping with what is already known about the importance of building a good therapeutic relationship, non-problem talk allows the therapist to get to know the person apart from the problems. For people with learning disabilities and/or autism, talking about things they like, things they do well or special interests usually gives the therapist access to many coping skills, significant abilities and strengths on which future solutions can be built. It also gives the therapist some insight into times when the problems for which the person was referred are not so problematic in the person's life.

(3) Best hopes for the session: again, the therapist learns from the client what it is he or she wants to be different as a result of coming to the therapy session on that day. This is in contrast to the therapist setting the goals for the session, perhaps in terms of talking about the person's thoughts or feelings. Instead, the client gets to say how he or she thinks the session has been useful. People with learning disabilities often say they want to

just talk, and that they want the therapist to listen. In terms of how they know whether or not the therapist is listening, clients often say if the therapist uses the client's words or writes things down, then he/she knows the therapist is listening.

(4) Preferred future: in strict SFBT terms, the 'miracle question' is used within the first session to structure discussion around what the person's life would be like without the problems that brought him or her to therapy. In terms of working with people who have learning disabilities or autism, it can be difficult for them to 'pretend' or 'imagine' a future at all, let alone a future without the problems they are having. However, people with cognitive disabilities are often able to describe a routine day in detail, starting with when and how they wake in the morning, then review that day with prompts from the therapist in terms of what might be different if they had the future they wanted. This gives the therapist information about how the desired changes will show up in the client's daily life. By highlighting the detail of how life will be different without the problem, it is more likely that the client or carers will actually notice the positive changes when they occur.

(5) Coping/exception questions: throughout discussion with the client, the solution-focused therapist will be wondering how the person has coped with the difficulties, who has noticed the person coping and asking about the times when the problem is not happening. This is based on the assumption that problems do not happen all the time, and identifying the detail of what is happening when things are going well. This leads to fascinating discussions with people who have histories of being marginalised, institutionalised, abused or neglected. The therapist may often be left wondering how a person who has been through such traumas has managed to turn out to be a funny, caring, eager to please individual instead of a homicidal maniac. Talking in detail about coping skills usually results in an overflow of client competencies, strengths and creativity. Identifying exceptions to the problem also helps to uncover things within the person's environment that help to lessen the impact of the problem.

(6) Scales: typically scales of 0 to 10 are used with 10 representing the best of something and 0 being the worst. If the person is able to relate to this way of thinking, scales can be used to bridge the understanding between client and therapist. Sometimes people with learning disabilities struggle with the idea of numbers and abstract concepts of 'better' and 'worse' so there are times when scales cannot be used effectively. However, scales lend themselves easily to modification. For example, a large square could be used to mean 'most' or 'best' or 'biggest' whilst a small square could be used to mean the opposite. Also, faces showing various emotions can be used to indicate positive and negative aspects of a scale. Once a position on the scale has been identified, work can begin identifying the detail of what one step higher on the scale would look like, as well as

highlighting the skills that have kept the person from being lower down on the scale.

(7) Feedback and ending: some solution-focused therapists take a break near the end of the session to leave the room and gather their thoughts about what they have heard. Very fortunate therapists have colleagues who have been observing the session and they can use this break to gather comments and ideas from them. Upon returning to the client, the idea is for the therapist to summarise what he or she understands to be the best hopes of the person as well as the strengths he or she has noticed which give the therapist hope that positive changes will occur.

(8) Task setting: occasionally a therapist will make a suggestion that the client might like to 'experiment' between sessions just to see what happens. Such an experiment might be that the person pretends his or her problems have gone away and behaves 'as if' he/she is in a good mood just to see what difference that makes to his/her carers. It is equally likely, however, that no between-session tasks will be suggested.

(9) Next appointment? Unlike some other therapies, solution-focused therapists usually ask clients whether or not they want to see them again. If they do, as often is the case with people who have learning disabilities, they are asked to decide how long they would like to wait before returning. Usually people with learning disabilities do not elect to return to therapy on a weekly basis. An interval of 2 to 4 weeks is generally preferred.

There has been little research into using SFBT with people who have cognitive impairment, although there is a rapidly growing body of research using the approach with other populations and with a wide variety of issues. Rhodes (2000) used the principles of SFBT when consulting with carers eight times over 6 months, resulting in a significant reduction in antisocial behaviour. Stoddart et al. (2001) found success using a modified version of SFBT with individuals who had mild learning disabilities, were self-referred and were supported in the therapeutic process by others. Skirrow (pers. comm.) used a solution-focused approach to interview six individuals recently discharged from psychology services to identify whether therapy had helped and if so how. The social validity of therapeutic interventions was discussed. Finally Saxby (pers. comm) used SFBT in first session interviews with families who had a child with learning disabilities. She found that SFBT highlighted the existing skills of parents and that interventions were ecologically sound in as much as they did not add to the already busy nature of parents' lives. The story of Mark illustrates the application of SFBT to a person with learning disabilities and mental health problems.

Mark was a 24 year old referred to the community team for adults with learning disabilities by the probation service. He had been arrested and charged with a public disorder offence and was now on probation. Mark was at risk of re-offending, and his parents indicated high levels of concern and stress as the main carer. Mark agreed that the first meeting could take place with his family as well as the probation officer.

Mark's family remarked on feeling a little less stressed between the time the appointment was made and the time of the first meeting. It turned out that even the promise of more support for their son and themselves gave them hope which in turn decreased the feeling of stress. Mark and the probation officer noted no pre-session improvement. In terms of how the family would know if the meeting was worthwhile, they identified two things. First they wanted to know how to respond to what they saw as Mark's oppositional behaviour and second they wanted reassurance that Mark would have some source of positive support besides themselves. The probation officer wanted to know whether or not the therapist felt Mark needed on-going psychotherapy in order to avoid re-offending. Mark could not think of any outcomes from the meeting that would make him think it had been worthwhile.

The gist of the miracle question revealed that if the present problems disappeared the family would be happy that Mark was living in his own flat, had friends who would not take advantage of him, had a job and was happy with his life. The probation officer said that Mark needed to attend all scheduled sessions, give better eye contact and talk more spontaneously during their meetings. Mark surprisingly warmed to the miracle question and described a day when he 'woke up with a lady beside him' and 'made her breakfast' then 'went off to his job as a joiner' sharing a lift with his mate. He even described the things he and his mate might talk about on the way to work.

The group became involved in identifying characteristics of Mark that made them hopeful he could achieve the life he described. Mark's eye contact with members of the group noticeably increased during this discussion. As often is the case, the list of positive attributes, skills, coping mechanisms, strengths and so on was very long indeed and filled the remainder of the first session. Mark opted to return for another appointment on his own, with the proviso that the family and probation officer could ring the therapist if they felt a need to.

Mark and the therapist met a further three times. The most important thing Mark decided was learning how to be friends with people who would not take advantage of him. By the fourth session, he had returned to a job he had previously held and was working his way back up to full time employment. He continued to be unsure how to make friends though he reported that he was talking more to people at work.

Several months later, the probation officer again made contact with the therapist to report that Mark was in full time employment and had moved into his own flat. He also had a girlfriend, who unfortunately had taken most of Mark's money before she left him. The probation officer said Mark had agreed to meet with the therapist again. Mark arrived at the office looking much the same as he had for the first meeting, with very little eye contact and stooped posture. He was very quiet initially, but as questions were asked about how he had managed to cope with work and a move to his own flat, his eye contact gradually increased. The therapist did not mention Mark's financial difficulties or his choice in girlfriends and Mark did not volunteer any information about these. His best hopes for the session were 'just to talk' and by the end of the meeting he said he felt better. He asked to come back in 2 weeks time. Mark and his therapist had a further four meetings during which they discussed how to tell if a person was a genuine friend or not. The therapist did not tell Mark how to do this, but listened to how Mark already made decisions and choices and together they tried to apply this to the way he made friends. Mark chose not to return to therapy, having had eight meetings in total, but occasionally he and the therapist connect briefly with text messages.

Throughout the eight meetings, the things that Mark had done 'wrong' were mentioned only in the context of talking about a future when things were better. No details were taken about the history of offending behaviour, about money mismanagement or about poor choices in friends. The discussions focused on the thousands of things Mark did right in his daily life, and moved at his pace using his language towards a future that he described. At the end of therapy, Mark said he had been helped, and identified some things that he was doing differently as a result of his meetings with the therapist. There was no further contact with the family after the first meeting, and only three phone conversations with the probation officer.

Emerging models of psychosocial intervention

Reminiscence

There is an emerging body of evidence regarding the use of reminiscence in older people with dementia. Reminiscence is seen as a positive activity, where a therapist can facilitate the discussion of the events and experiences of the past. The focus of simple reminiscence is on providing pleasure, communication and socialisation. Baro (2002) suggests that this can take the form of an individual or group approach, structured or free flowing, spontaneous or prompted, general or specific. Reminiscence can also be conducted using the medium of life story work, which will help to provide value and understanding of the person's network of friends and relatives, activities and achievements. This will also help to formulate care plans based on personalised interactions. Use of reminiscence with people with Down's syndrome and older people with learning disabilities needs to be fully explored in order to understand its practicalities and evaluation.

Life story work

People with learning disabilities experience emotions (both good and bad) as any other person does, and most people have memories of the past, their relationships and friends, emotionally turbulent times and phases in their life and feelings of loss. According to Hussain and Raczka (1997), life story work involves gathering a variety of information on all aspects of the person's life, from personal experiences, feelings and thoughts on life changes, families and relationships, to more factual information on birthdays, schools, homes lived in and so on. They suggest that life story work is not the creation of a complete life story but should highlight certain aspects of people's lives, thus improving our understanding of the way in which people with learning disabilities perceive everyday events and interactions.

   Life story work can allow people to examine their own feelings and experiences and hence this needs to be conducted with utmost sensitivity and professional integrity. Life story work enables people with learning disability to identify their own feelings relating to people and places and this needs to be channelled effectively to help people resolve conflicts and dilemmas. It helps people to examine past experiences and events and can help to facilitate reflection and positive emotional well-being. For people with learning disabilities, life story work has applications in bereavement counselling (Read et al. 1999), for boosting self-esteem and confidence building, and in making choices and decisions about present and future lives.

Helping models

An holistic approach to people with learning disabilities and mental health disorders should not be limited to the use of just cognitive, behaviour or psychodynamic therapies. Holistic care is multi-dimensional because of the range of helping models provided for these individuals by their family carers or nurses. For example a person with learning disability and anxiety living in a group home may receive help and support from nurses and other professionals. This may involve anxiety management training at home, whilst going shopping or engaging in any other outdoor pursuits or entertainments. The nurses helping and supporting this person will be involved in engaging the person in a range of activities such as personal care, socialisation, skills facilitation and development, friendship and relationship building, to mention a few of the caring activities. Whilst helping the person to manage anxiety at home and outside, it is important that nurses and other carers are able to identify and record the intricate processes involved in helping the person on a daily basis. The careful documentation and articulation of the caring processes will help the person with learning disabilities and others to visualise the helping models adopted for the therapeutic care. This will also help clinicians to identify the factors contributing to the outcome of interventions.

The helping models adopted in the holistic care of each individual tell a unique story. The conceptualisation of helping models for each individual may very well involve established therapeutic approaches such as cognitive or behaviour therapy, but most importantly it will help to identify essential caring processes by nurses. The focus on helping models will help us to understand the spectrum of care processes involved in holistic care. This may help nurses and other professionals to see the person as a whole and not in terms of the symptoms or behaviours shown by the person.

Conclusion

In this chapter we have seen the application of psychosocial interventions for people with learning disabilities with behaviour and mental health disorders. The evidence base of the various psychosocial interventions is limited and further evaluation of the various approaches is necessary. There is an urgent need for the development of practice-based evidence models that may help to highlight the factors contributing to the long-term sustainability of these interventions.

References

Baro, F. (2002) Psychosocial interventions for dementia: a review. In: M. Maj and N. Sartorius (Eds) *Dementia*. Chichester: John Wiley.

Beail, N. (1998) Psychoanalytic psychotherapy with men with intellectual disabilities: a preliminary outcome study. *British Journal of Medical Psychology*, **71**, 1–11.

Beail, N. and Warden, S. (1996) Evaluation of a psychodynamic psychotherapy with intellectual disabilities: rational, design and preliminary outcome data. *Journal of Applied Research in Intellectual Disabilities*, **9**, 223–228.

Beck, A.T. (1967) *Depression: Causes and Treatment*. Philadelphia: University of Pennsylvania Press.

Benson, B.A. (1986) Anger management training. *Psychiatric Aspects of Mental Retardation Reviews*, **5**, 51–55.

Benson, B.A. and Havercamp, S.M. (1999) Behavioural approaches to treatment: principles and practices. In: N. Bouras (Ed.) *Psychiatric and Behavioural Disorders in Developmental Disabilities and Mental Retardation*. Cambridge: Cambridge University Press.

Bernstein, D.A. and Borkovec, T.D. (1973) *Progressive Relaxation Training: A Manual for the Helping Professions*. Champaign: Research Press.

Berry, P. (2003) Psychodynamic therapy and intellectual disabilities: dealing with challenging behaviour. *International Journal of Disability, Development and Education*, **50**, 39–51.

Black, L., Cullen, C. and ·Novaco, R. (1997) Anger assessment for people with mild learning disabilities in secure settings. In: B. Stenfert Kroese, D. Dagnan and K. Loumidis (Eds) *Cognitive-Behaviour Therapy for People with Learning Disabilities*. London: Routledge.

Bliss, E.V. (2002) Integrative Solution Focused Brief Therapy Case Study: Essay for SFBT Course, Birmingham. clarks@globalnet.co.uk.

Brown, D. and Pedder, J. (1991) *Introduction to Psychotherapy*, 2nd edition. London: Tavistock/Routledge.

Calamari, J.E., Geist, G.O. and Shahbazian, M.J. (1987) Evaluation of multiple component relaxation training with developmentally disabled persons. *Research in Developmental Disabilities*, **8**, 55–70.

Dagnan, D. and Chadwick, P. (1997) Cognitive-behaviour therapy for people with learning disabilities: assessment and intervention. In: B. Stenfert Kroese, D. Dagnan and K. Loumidis (Eds) *Cognitive-Behaviour Therapy for People with Learning Disabilities*. London: Routledge.

De Groef, J. and Heinemann, E. (1999) *Psychoanalysis and Mental Handicap*. London: Free Association Press.

Department of Health (2001) *Treatment Choice in Psychological Therapies and Counselling – Evidence Based Clinical Practice Guideline*. London: Department of Health.

De Shazer, S., Berg, I.F., Lipchik, E., et al. (1986) Brief therapy: focussed solution development. *Family Process*, **25**, 207–221.

Dixon, M.S. and Gunary, R.M. (1986) Fear of dogs: group treatment of people with mental handicaps. *Mental Handicap*, **14**, 6–9.

Dobson, K.S. and Dozois, D.J. (2001) Historical and philosophical bases of the cognitive behavioural therapies. In: K.S. Dobson (Ed.) *Handbook of Cognitive Behavioural Therapies*. New York: The Guilford Press.

Ellis, A. (1962) *Reason and Emotion in Psychotherapy*. New York: Stewart.

Frankish, P. (1992) A psychodynamic approach to emotional difficulties with a social framework. *Journal of Intellectual Disability Research*, **36**, 559–563.

Helsel, W.J. and Matson, J.L. (1988) The relationship of depression to social skills and intellectual functioning in mentally retarded adults. *Journal of Mental Deficiency Research*, **32**, 411–418.

Hollins, S. (2001) Psychotherapeutic methods. In: A. Dosen and K. Day (Eds) *Treating Mental Illness and Behaviour Disorders in Children and Adults with Mental Retardation*. Washington DC: American Psychiatric Press.

Hollins, S. (2003) Counselling and psychotherapy in seminars in the psychiatry of learning disabilities. In: W. Fraser and M. Kerr (Eds) *Seminars in the Psychiatry of Learning Disabilities*. London: Gaskell Press.

Hussain, F. and Raczka, R. (1997) Life story work for people with learning disabilities. *British Journal of Learning Disabilities*, **25**, 73–76.

Iveson, C. (2002) Solution-focussed brief therapy. *Advances in Psychiatric Treatment*, **8**, 149–157.

Jacobson, E. (1929) *Progressive Relaxation*. Chicago: University of Chicago Press.

Laman, D.S. and Reiss, S. (1987) Social skill deficiencies associated with depressed mood of mentally retarded adults. *American Journal of Mental Deficiency*, **92**, 224–229.

Legget, J., Hurn, C. and Goodman, W. (1997) Teaching psychological strategies for managing auditory hallucinations. A case report. *British Journal of Learning Disabilities*, **25**, 158–161.

Lindsay, W. and Baty, F. (1986) Behavioural relaxation training: explorations with adults who are mentally handicapped. *Mental Handicap*, **14**, 160–162.

Lindsay, W. Michie, A., Baty, F. and McKenzie, K. (1988) Dog phobia in people with mental handicaps: anxiety management training and exposure treatments. *Mental Handicap Research*, **1**, 39–48.

Lindsay, W., Baty, F., Michie, A. and Richardson, I. (1989) A comparison of anxiety treatments with adults who have moderate and severe mental retardation. *Research in Developmental Disabilities*, **10**, 129–140.

Lindsay, W.R., Howells, L. and Pitcaithly, P. (1993) Cognitive therapy for depression with individuals with intellectual disabilities. *British Journal of Medical Psychology*, **66**, 135–141.

Lindsay, W., Neilson, C. and Lawrenson, H. (1997) Cognitive-behaviour therapy for anxiety in people with learning disabilities. In: B. Stenfert Kroese, D. Dagnan and K. Loumidis (Eds) *Cognitive-Behaviour Therapy for People with Learning Disabilities*. London: Routledge.

Lindsay, W., Overend, H., Allan, R. and Williams, C. (1998) Using specific approaches for individual problems in the management of anger and aggression. *British Journal of Learning Disabilities*, **26**, 44–50.

Matson, J.L., Smiroldo, B.B. and Bamburg, J.W. (1998) The relationship of social skills to psychopathology for individuals with severe or profound mental retardation. *Journal of Intellectual and Developmental Disability*, **23**, 137–145.

Moore, E., Adams, R., Elsworth, J. and Lewis, J. (1997) An anger management group for people with a learning disability. *British Journal of Learning Disabilities*, **25**, 53–57.

Novaco, R.W. (1975) *Anger Control: The Development and Evaluation of an experimental treatment*. Lexington, Massachusetts: D.C. Heath.

Prout, H.T. and Nowak-Drabik, K.M. (2003) Psychotherapy with persons who have mental retardation: an evaluation of effectiveness. *American Journal on Mental Retardation*, **108**, 82–93.

Read, S., Messenger, N. and Oats, S. (1999) Bereavement counselling and support for people with a learning disability: identifying issues and exploring possibilities. *British Journal of Learning Disabilities*, **27**, 99–104.

Rhodes, J. (2000) Solution-focused consultation in a residential setting. *Clinical Psychology Forum*, **141**, 29–33.

Rose, J., West, C. and Clifford, D. (2000) Group interventions for anger in people with intellectual disabilities. *Research in Developmental Disabilities*, **12**, 211–224.

Royal College of Psychiatrists (2004) *Psychotherapy and Learning Disability*. Council Report CR116. London: Royal College of Psychiatrists.

Sinason, V. (1992) *Mental Handicap and the Human Condition*. London: Free Association Books.

Stenfert Kroese, B. (1997) Cognitive-behaviour therapy for people with learning disabilities: conceptual and contextual issues. In: B. Stenfert Kroese, D. Dagnan and K. Loumidis (Eds) *Cognitive-Behaviour Therapy for People with Learning Disabilities*. London: Routledge.

Stoddart, K., McDonnell, J., Temple, V. and Mustata, A. (2001) Is brief better? A modified brief solution-focused therapy approach for adults with a developmental delay. *Journal of Systemic Therapy*, **20**, 24–40.

Storr, A. (1979) *The Art of Psychotherapy*. Oxford: Oxford University Press.

Strupp, H.H. (1978) Psychotherapy research and practice: an overview. In: S. Garfield and A. Bergin (Eds) *Handbook of Psychotherapy and Behaviour Change*. New York: Wiley.

Waitman, A. and Conboy-Hill, S. (1992) *Psychotherapy and Mental Hnadicap*. London: Sage.

Willner, P., Jones, J., Tams, R. and Green, G. (2002) A randomised controlled trial of the efficiency of a cognitive-behavioural anger management group for clients with learning disabilities. *Journal of Applied Research in Intellectual Disabilities*, **15**, 224–235.

Wolpe, J. (1958) *Psychotherapy by Reciprocal Inhibition*. Stanford, California: Stanford University Press.

Further reading

Bliss, E.V. (2004) *The Missing Link Support Service*. clarks@globalnet.co.uk.
Sharry, J. (2001) *Solution-Focussed Group Work*. London: Sage.

Chapter 9

Professional and legal issues

In the process of caring we need to observe professional codes of conduct and legal frameworks that govern our day-to-day practice with vulnerable individuals. This chapter will explore the themes of capacity to give consent for assessment and treatment, professional codes of conduct and the duty of care. The Mental Health Act 1983 and its application to people with learning disabilities will be discussed. The theme of risk and risk assessment will also be explored in the context of offending behaviour.

Key themes

- Consent and issues of consent with people with learning disabilities
- The duty of care and professionalism
- Mental health legislation
- Forensic aspects
- Risk assessment

Introduction

Over the last four decades the care of people with learning disabilities has experienced a significant paradigm shift. In Britain in the 1960s and 1970s most people with learning disabilities were living in long-stay institutions and subjected to a custodial regime of care dominated by the medical profession (Ryan and Thomas 1995). These decades saw a number of enquiries into the care of people living within these institutions (Howe Report 1969; Fisher et al. 1978). Work by Goffman (1961), Wolfensberger (1972) and Oswin (1978) further highlighted the plight of adults and children living in such contained environments, discussing and propounding concepts such as institutionalisation and normalisation.

Institutional practices such as rigidity of routine, block treatment of people and depersonalisation frequently eroded all sense of well-being, self-esteem, skills and confidence. People living within such institutions were often unable or discouraged to make decisions about their daily life, what clothes they wore and what to eat, as the large organisation churned out activities, social events, food and clothing.

Various reports published over the remaining years of the 20th century (DHSS 1971; King's Fund Centre 1980) made various attempts to address issues of personal freedom, 'ordinary life' and autonomy, these being influenced by the philosophy of normalisation (Nirje 1969; Wolfensberger 1972; O'Brien and Tyne 1981) and the growing movement of human rights, commencing with the *Universal Declaration of Human Rights* (United Nations 1948), the *Declaration of the General and Specific Rights of the Mentally Retarded* (United Nations 1971) and culminating in the Human Rights Act (1998) and the recent Mental Capacity Act.

The concept of the individual's right to self-determination underpins the above legislation. Case law in England and Wales has established that people who are competent have the right to determine whether to accept medical treatment or not. If competent individuals refuse to give consent for treatment of a physical disorder, this *must* be respected even if it is likely to lead to their death. This, however, does not apply to the treatment of mental disorder. Mental health legislation in England and Wales under specified circumstances allows compulsory admission and treatment of individuals with mental disorders even if they have the capacity to make the necessary treatment decision and decide not to accept the treatment recommended.

It is now usually accepted that people with learning disabilities have the right to make decisions, choices and give consent when able regarding all aspects of their lives, such as whether to partake in community activities, develop their skills, which diet to follow and which medication to take. The Mental Capacity Act suggests the following statement of principles:

- Every adult has the right to make his/her own decisions and must be assumed to have the capacity to do so unless it is proved otherwise.
- Everyone should be encouraged and enabled to make his/her own decisions, or to participate as fully as possible in decision-making, by being given the help and support needed to make and express a choice.
- Individuals must retain the right to make what might be seen as eccentric or unwise decisions.
- Decisions made on behalf of people without capacity should be made in their best interests, giving priority to achieving what they themselves would have wanted.
- Decisions made on behalf of someone else should be those that are least restrictive to their basic rights and freedoms.

Holland (2003) highlights that people's decisions are influenced by the circumstances in which they find themselves, as well as by their values, beliefs, morals, social backgrounds and experiences. Some people by virtue of having a mental disability, intellectual disability or head injury may have difficulties in making decisions. For some people with learning disabilities the influence of family or paid carers may impinge upon their ability to make or carry through their own decisions.

Consider the following scenarios. Are there any issues regarding choices, decisions or consent?

Scenario 1: Ken has severe learning disabilities; he has no verbal communication and has very limited self-help skills. He begins to head bang, an unusual behaviour for him, and refuses to eat. After a few days his face is swelling on the jaw line and it is obvious he has an abscess under one of his teeth. When nurses approach him he lashes out and curls into a ball. He needs dental treatment.

Scenario 2: Martha moved out of a long-stay institution in 1981 and now lives alone and manages all her own affairs; she periodically believes her neighbours are spying on her and this leads to her being verbally abusive towards anyone in her vicinity. She is overweight, has high blood pressure and diabetes. She has been prescribed tablets to reduce her blood pressure and blood glucose but she refuses to take them. She also refuses to see psychiatrists and does not believe she has a problem.

Scenario 3: Freda aged 24 years has moderate learning disabilities and lives at home with her mother who cares for her. She has recently started a relationship with a young man and her mother has taken her to the health centre in order for her to be given the contraceptive pill.

Scenario 4: Stephen has a moderate learning disability and mental health problem and lives in a small group home. He has recently become agitated, accusing other residents of hiding his things and the staff of trying to poison him with his tablets. He is increasingly becoming both verbally and physically abusive, making the others who live in the group home and staff fearful of what he may do.

Scenario 5: Jane has learning disabilities and lives in a 12-bedded mental health unit. Jane is subject to Section 3 of the Mental Health Act for treatment. She sometimes refuses to dress in the morning and walks around the unit naked.

It should not be assumed that a person with learning disability is not able to make a decision or express personal choice with appropriate support. Similarly a person with a mental health problem cannot be assumed to be incompetent of making treatment choices merely on the basis of a diagnosed illness. Just because someone has a learning disability and mental health needs it should not be assumed that he or she is unable to consent or make an informed decision. Therefore when addressing the care of a person with learning disabilities one should ensure as far as possible that the person understands and approves of actions being taken to help him or her, whether it is self-care, for example dressing, or carrying out extensive surgery. Not only is this an essential component of good practice but also it is a legal requirement. Failure to obtain consent is unethical and may lead to disciplinary action within the nursing profession, for example if you reveal information about a person without obtaining his/her consent (*Code of Professional Conduct*, Nursing and Midwifery Council 2002, Clause 5). Or if you perform an intimate bodily examination without consent it may well be regarded as common assault, leading to prosecution, or claims for damages, or both.

Therefore, before deciding to intervene with anyone in the above scenarios one needs to remember the basic precept that every adult has the right to make a decision unless proved otherwise.

However, with the above scenarios there are a number of questions that you may have asked yourself: is Ken capable of making the decision, as he is obviously in pain but seems to be refusing further help? Does Martha realise the consequences of not taking her medication? Has she received enough information and understood this for her to be fully aware of the implications of her decision? Is Freda acting under pressure from her mother? Is Stephen aware of his own actions?

According to the Department of Health (2001a), for a person's consent to be valid, three conditions have to be met:

(1) The person must be capable of making that particular decision.
(2) The person must be acting voluntarily, that is he/she should be making the decision freely without coercion or external pressure.
(3) The person must be provided with enough information to enable him/her to make the decision.

The key issues in deciding whether an individual has the capacity to make a treatment decision are the ability to: communicate a choice; understand, believe and retain the relevant information; and balance the information in order to arrive at a choice. In law, any individual is presumed to have the capacity to make a treatment decision unless proven otherwise as outlined below:

• If the person is unable to take in and retain the information relevant to the decision, especially the likely consequences of having or not having the treatment.
• If the person is unable to believe the information.
• If the person is unable to weigh the information in the balance as part of a process of arriving at the decision.

For a person with learning disabilities it is important to try to maximise the person's capacity to make decisions by using simple language and non-verbal, visual materials, for example photos, videos or drawings. Information should be presented in small amounts and repeated frequently. Adequate time should be available in a safe, familiar environment with an advocate or familiar carer being present. It is important to encourage the person to ask questions and to give him or her an information sheet about the proposed treatment, which is written in simple language with bullet points and additional appropriate pictorial information.

Some decisions may be less complex, for example whether to take 'iron tablets' for anaemia, whereas other decisions are more complex with the person requiring understanding of alternative choices with differing outcomes, such as whether to undergo a hysterectomy or not. As Gunn (1994) indicates, capacity and incapacity are the ends of a continuum; there are degrees of capacity. From a legal perspective, however, capacity is dichotomous, that is either one has capacity or one does not have it. Thus this poses difficulties in some clinical scenarios where it may be difficult to say for certain whether the person has capacity or not. At times further clarification from the High Court may be required.

Fovargue and Keywood (2000) demonstrated that participation in health care decisions frequently did not depend fully upon someone's capacity to make decisions but on the perspectives and motivation of the people caring for the person. Family members or care professionals in this study unduly influenced many of those who took part in the research. It quickly becomes apparent that people with learning disabilities require information about different interventions, the consequences of interventions and their behaviour. The NHS Executive (1998) states that information must be provided in suitable formats in appropriate ways that take into account the level of learning disabilities, sensory impairments and languages in use.

In order to effectively provide information to people with learning disabilities it is imperative that carers are aware of the cognitive (thinking and problem solving) ability of the person to whom they are imparting information. It is inappropriate to use written information if the person is unable to read and it is futile to use symbols when the person is unable to comprehend two-dimensional figures. The White Paper *Valuing People* (Department of Health 2001b) and other policy documents (Department of Health 2002) highlight and advocate the partnership model of care delivery in a multi-agency and multi-professional framework. As a result, it is important to ensure that someone's level of comprehension is recorded (Nursing and Midwifery Council 1998a) so that all staff are aware of the person's needs when making decisions.

Sometimes all the person may require to assimilate the information is for the professional to go through the information simply and coherently, answer any questions the person with learning disabilities has and give him or her the opportunity and time to work through the issues. A person should not be regarded as incapable of doing so merely because the decisions reached appear to others to be unwise or irrational. Everyone uses a different belief or value system, so even if the decision appears irrational, as long as they understand what is involved in that decision, carers should abide by that person's decision. For example, if someone has agoraphobia he or she may well refuse to participate in community activities or if someone has a gangrenous foot and refuses to undergo surgery as he/she says he/she would rather be dead than live without a leg, that person is demonstrating some understanding of the consequences of his/her actions.

If Martha had originally agreed to the medication but then refuses to take it, what is the position? As with everyone people are allowed to change their mind if they have the capacity to do so, and conversely Martha may decide to take the medication she originally refused. Therefore as carers one has a duty to ensure that people with learning disabilities are aware that their decisions do not have to be binding and that they can change their mind at any time and reverse their decision. Even if someone is unable to make a decision or consent to treatment as in the scenario of Stephen, it does not mean that person will always be incapable of making that decision. Therefore, assessment of capacity needs to be reassessed regularly over time.

Nurses can be said to have a 'duty of care' to ensure that no harm occurs to the person either by their action or by their inaction. For example, in the scenario of Stephen, if a nurse approaches and he says, 'Go away, I don't want you to come near me', the nurse may well literally interpret that as 'Do not approach me' and 'Leave me alone'; but it could be argued that Stephen is not fully exercising informed consent and does not fully understand or appreciate what the nurse is about to do. One could therefore expect a competent nurse to briefly explain his/her purpose and reiterate to Stephen his option not to be subjected to a nursing intervention. If Stephen still does not want the nurse near him then the nurse would have to respect his decision and make another attempt to work with him later. However, if Stephen's behaviour poses a risk to himself or others then the nurse has to intervene.

The Nursing and Midwifery Council (1998b) clearly states:

'Nurses need to understand their duty of care to clients. This duty is dependent on the context of the care and the consequences of clients' behaviour on themselves and those around them. Your actions will be assessed according to whether they were reasonable under the circumstances. It is important to ensure that a range of alternatives is explored.'

Nevertheless, there will be some occasions when information has been presented in simple terms but the person is still unable to make a decision on the matter in question. The person is then said to be without capacity to make the treatment decision. However, it is still possible for someone to lawfully provide treatment and care. This may be true of Ken and Jane in the scenarios above. Ken is obviously in a great deal of pain but is unable to communicate his needs or desires to his carers and Jane seems unable to understand the consequences of her actions.

Issues of capacity are further complicated when the person has learning disabilities and mental health needs as in the case of Stephen. However, before you finally decide that the person is unable to make the decision, you must ensure that you have done all that you can to inform the person and elicit a decision from them.

A nurse must substantiate future conduct by recording in detail what has been said to the person and his or her reactions in order to demonstrate a reasoned and systematic approach to care (Nursing and Midwifery Council 2002). In other words nurses must demonstrate their accountability, that is, explain how they have arrived at that particular course of action and should accept the responsibility for their actions as well. The *Code of Professional Conduct* (Nursing and Midwifery Council 2002) clearly states that nurses must respect the individuality of people in their care (Clause 2). Jane is behaving in an unacceptable manner and she needs to be helped to understand that undressing in public is not appropriate, and why this is so. In some incidences medication may be given compulsorily or if Jane continues to refuse to put on clothes she may be contained in her room in order to ensure that she does not place herself in a further vulnerable position. In this scenario the symptom of Jane's mental health condition is seen to be so severe then it overrides her personal wishes.

Sometimes it may be useful to discuss the person's needs with someone who is close to the person, such as a relative. That person cannot consent to medical treatment for Ken but he or she will be able to discuss and aid any decision-making based on the best interest of the person. In Ken's situation it would be poor care or neglect if carers were to leave him in such distress and pain; therefore one could say it is in Ken's best interests to receive dental treatment. However, one would expect carers, parents, close relatives and dental staff to discuss the options and method of treatment, although legally the final decision should be that of the health professionals as they are the ones responsible for Ken's care.

However, what does 'best interests' mean? According to the Department of Health (2001a) best interests are more than medical benefits. Issues such as general well-being, relationships and welfare should be taken into account. It should also be remembered that even when people lack capacity to consent they might still be able to express their willingness or not to co-operate with the care or treatment being offered. These indications should always be responded to and acted upon; for example, if someone needs medication for mental ill health and becomes distressed at taking tablets then other methods of administration should be considered such as liquid form.

When deciding upon the best interests of the person with learning disabilities the needs of the family most likely will be interwoven, but the focus should be on the person. Therefore, if Freda's mother wants her to take the contraceptive pill as it would protect her from unwanted pregnancy, this is not in itself a valid reason for Freda to take the pill. Freda needs to also understand what other forms of contraception are available and the consequences of not using contraception adequately.

Consent: the basic principles

Consent is the voluntary and continuing permission to receive a particular treatment, based on an adequate knowledge of the purpose, nature, likely effects

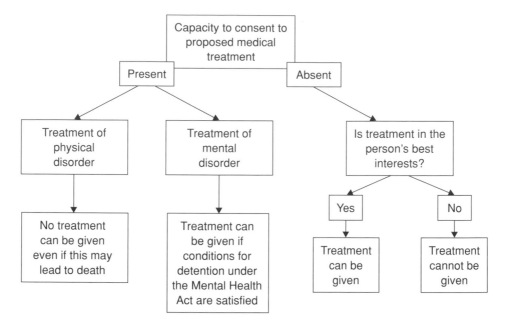

Fig. 9.1 Admission for assessment and treatment – issues of information and consent.

and risks of that treatment including the likelihood of its success and alternatives to it. Permission given under any unfair or undue pressure is not 'consent'. Mental disorder by itself does not make a patient incapable of giving or refusing consent (Fig. 9.1). People who are unable to give informed consent may fall into the following categories:

- Those without capacity to consent:
    - *An immature child*: a parent or person with parental responsibility may consent.
    - *An unconscious patient*: the patient may be treated if there is an urgent need to preserve life, health or well-being, unless unequivocal, reliable evidence is provided to show that the patient did not want treatment.
    - A patient who lacks capacity but is in need of medical care that is '*in the patient's best interests*' may be treated without consent.
- Adults who are not competent to give consent: no-one can give consent on behalf of an incompetent adult. Treatment can be undertaken if it is in the 'best interest' of the person. 'Best interests' include factors such as the wishes and beliefs of the patient when competent, his or her current wishes, general well-being, and spiritual and religious welfare. Where a person has never been competent, relatives, carers and friends may be best placed to advise on the person's needs and preferences.

The *Bournewood judgment* is based on a court case concerning a 48-year-old man with autism (Mr. L) [*R. v Bournewood and Mental Health NHS Trust ex parte*

L (1998 All ER 319)]. Mr. L was a resident at a hospital run by Bournewood NHS Trust. Mr. L was unable to speak. As part of the resettlement, he went to live with a couple who were his carers. They regarded him as one of the family. One day at a day centre Mr. L became agitated. As his carers could not be contacted, Mr. L was given a sedative and taken to hospital. The doctor decided that there was no need to detain Mr. L in hospital under the Mental Health Act as he was compliant and did not resist or attempt to run away. He was kept in hospital on an informal basis. His carers were not allowed to see him for nearly 4 months. They demanded his release but had no statutory basis to challenge the doctor's decision. The carers took action against the Trust, claiming that he was unlawfully detained. (See Kramer 2002 for more details of the case.)

It was deemed that, if at the time of admission, the patient is mentally incapable of consent, but does not object to entering hospital and receiving care or treatment, then admission should be informal. The *common law doctrine of necessity* states that the treatment must be:

- Necessary to save life or prevent a deterioration or ensure an improvement in the patient's physical or mental health; and
- In accordance with the practice accepted at the time by a reasonable body of medical opinion skilled in the particular form of treatment.

An exception to the above rule is the procedure of sterilisation where the approval of the High Court should be sought by way of a declaration.

The delivery of all mental health services is now guided by the care programme approach (CPA), which is discussed in the context of service provision in Chapter 10. Care management, which was previously a responsibility of social services, is now integrated within the CPA. Thus any professional within the multidisciplinary community mental health team including the social worker can be the care coordinator under the CPA. The case example of John highlights the difficulties faced by John's care staff at home and his admission to hospital.

John is a 52-year-old man with severe learning disabilities with a well documented history of bipolar affective disorder. His behaviour had deteriorated 6 weeks prior to admission to hospital. He was becoming increasingly difficult to manage at the group home, particularly at night. He was awake throughout the night and extremely restless. He was undressing, going out into the garden and even climbing over the garden fence. He was agitated and aggressive and had punched a member of staff. This was quite unlike John when he was well. He was initially managed at home by increasing the dose of his mood stabiliser and antipsychotic medication. Despite this he continued to deteriorate and his care staff could no longer safely manage him at home. Thus informal admission was arranged. John came into hospital willingly and was surprisingly cooperative on the acute general psychiatry ward. He had previously been admitted to the same unit and was thus familiar with ward routine and staff members. He had a single room and his care staff continued to support him daily while he was in hospital. His mental state improved with further medication changes in hospital and he was discharged back to his group home after a hospital stay of 4 weeks.

Covert administration of medicines

Under certain circumstances, for instance when a person with severe or profound learning disability who lacks capacity to make a treatment decision but needs to take medication, for example for an underactive thyroid, and refuses to do so, one may need to administer the medication in the person's best interests. The Nursing and Midwifery Council (NMC) recognises the importance of respecting an individual's autonomy when he or she decides to refuse medication; however, the NMC (2001) has produced a position statement on the covert administration of medicines. This was discussed at the Royal College of Nursing's annual congress in 2002 (www.rcn.org.uk/news/congress2002). There are times when a person with severe disability can neither consent nor refuse treatment. Treatment should, according to the NMC, be made available to such patients in accordance with the principles of best interests and administered in the least restrictive way.

The NMC further advises that in exceptional circumstances medicines may need to be administered within food with the patient unaware that this is being done. In such circumstances all efforts must be made to give medication openly in its normal tablet or syrup form. Consideration of the relevant legislation (the Mental Health Act in the UK and also Adults with Incapacity in Scotland) is important. There must also be clear expectation that the patient will benefit from such measures and that they will not result in any significant harm either mental or physical. The proposed treatment plan should be discussed with the nearest relative or nominated representative and included in the care plan. The GP should be informed in writing of such a plan. A clear record of reasons for deciding that the person does not have the capacity to consent to the proposed treatment must be recorded in the clinical notes. Regular reviews of the need to continue covert administration of medicines are important at multiprofessional meetings.

The Mental Health Act 1983

The Mental Health Act came into being in 1983 (Department of Health and Welsh Office 1983). The *Code of Practice* gives guidance on how the Act should be applied. A revised *Code of Practice* published in 1999 (Department of Health and Welsh Office 1999) pursuant to Section 118 of the Act takes into account case law and changes in practice and terminology.

The Code states that *impaired intellect* must be evaluated on the basis of reliable and careful assessment including usually a formal psychological assessment. The evidence of the degree and nature of social competence should be based on reliable and recent observations from a number of sources such as social workers, nurses and psychologists. Such evidence should include the results of one or more social functioning assessment tests, for example the adaptive behaviour scales (Nihira et al. 1974) or Vineland social maturity scale (Doll 1965). The Code of Practice advises that 'no patient should be classified under the Act as mentally impaired or severely mentally impaired without an assessment by a consultant psychiatrist in learning disabilities and a formal psychological assessment. Furthermore this assessment should be part of a complete assessment by medical, nursing, social work and psychology professionals with experience in learning disabilities, in consultation with a relative, friend or supporter of the patient'.

Mental disorder

The Mental Health Act divides mental disorder into four categories: mental illness, mental impairment, severe mental impairment and psychopathic disorder.

Mental illness

Mental illness is not defined further in the Act.

Mental impairment

Mental impairment is defined as a state of arrested or incomplete development of the mind, which includes significant impairment of intelligence and social functioning and is associated with abnormally aggressive behaviour or seriously irresponsible conduct.

Severe mental impairment

The difference between severe mental impairment and mental impairment is a matter of clinical judgement guided by current professional practice and includes incomplete or arrested development of mind which means that the disability present has permanently prevented the usual maturation of intellectual and social development. This excludes those in whom the learning disability occurred due to accident, injury or illness after a point usually accepted as complete development (age 18).

Psychopathic disorder

Psychopathic disorder is a persistent disorder or disability of the mind (with or without significant impairment of intelligence) resulting in abnormally aggressive behaviour or seriously irresponsible conduct.

Abnormally aggressive behaviour

Mental impairment or severe mental impairment also include abnormally aggressive behaviour or seriously irresponsible conduct. The former should be based on observations of behaviour in different settings leading to the conclusion that the behaviour problem is outside the usual range of aggressive behaviour and is causing actual damage and/or real distress. The behavioural problem is severe or persistent and recent.

Seriously irresponsible conduct is based on behavioural observations that show a lack of responsibility, a disregard for the consequences of actions, and 'which leads to actual damage or real distress, either recently or persistently or with excessive severity'.

The Code of Practice clarifies that a person with severe learning disabilities who lacks the capacity to make personal health decisions may be admitted to hospital voluntarily (on an informal basis), if he or she does not object to being in hospital. In this case the person's admission and care must be in his or her best interests and in accordance with the common law doctrine of necessity.

Under the Mental Health Act, there are three main groups of compulsory order for assessment and treatment:

(1)   Admission for assessment (Sections 2, 4, 5, 135 and 136)
(2)   Treatment orders (Sections 3 and 7)
(3)   Admission and transfer of patients who have committed criminal offences (Sections 37, 41, 47 and 49)

Admission for assessment

Section 2 of the Mental Health Act – application for admission for assessment
The following criteria must be satisfied:

- The patient is suffering from a mental disorder, which requires admission to hospital for further assessment or assessment followed by treatment.
- Admission is necessary in the interests of the patient's health *or* safety *or* for the protection of others.
- Application is made by an Approved Social Worker (ASW) or nearest relative.
- Recommendations are made by two doctors, one the patient's GP and the other a Section 12 approved doctor, usually a consultant psychiatrist or a staff grade doctor specialising in psychiatry.

The duration of Section 2 is 28 days and it cannot be renewed. The patient has a right of appeal to the Mental Health Review Tribunal (MHRT) within the first 14 days of the section. Discharge from this section can be authorised by the responsible medical officer (RMO), that is, the doctor in charge of the treatment, the person's nearest relative, hospital manager or the MHRT.

Section 4 – emergency order for assessment

This gives the power to detain a person in an emergency. It is usually completed by one doctor (preferably the GP) and occasionally is useful in the general hospital A&E department. It is only used when there is likely to be an undue delay in obtaining the opinion of a Section 12 approved doctor and such delay would adversely affect the patient's health. It is used only in emergencies when it is the intention to complete Section 2. The doctor is required to state the reasons why undue delay is expected in obtaining the second medical opinion and how long the delay may be.

The grounds are as for Section 2, that is, the person is suffering from a mental disorder that requires in-patient care and this is in the interests of their health *or* safety *or* for the protection of others. Application is made by approved Social Worker (ASW) or nearest relative. The duration of Section 4 is 72 hours, and it lapses unless converted to Section 2.

Section 5 – informal holding of patients already in hospital
Section 5/2 – holding power by doctor

This is an emergency measure to allow time to complete a Section 2 or 3 assessment. It allows detention of an in-patient for up to 72 hours. The application can be made by the RMO or a nominated deputy, usually the junior doctor on call. Patients retain their common law right to refuse treatment. It is bad practice to use this section more than once with the same patient within a short time period. Only the RMO can discharge the patient from this section. The case of Amy (see below) illustrates the application of Section 5/2.

Section 5/4 – holding power by nurse

A registered nurse (RMN or RNMH) may invoke this holding power. The nurse must record that the patient is suffering from a mental disorder and needs to be prevented from leaving the hospital in the interests of his or her health or safety or for the protection of others. This applies only when the patient is already under treatment for a mental disorder and the duty doctor is not immediately available. Duration of this order is 6 hours, but it lapses on arrival of the doctor, who then has to decide whether to detain the patient further under Section 5/2.

Section 135 – warrant searching for and removing patients who are in the community to a place of safety

In this case information must be provided on oath by an ASW to a justice of the peace or a magistrate. This power authorises the police to enter premises by force if necessary. This is applied for when there is reason to suspect that a person suffering from a mental disorder is unable to care for him- or herself or is being ill-treated or neglected. In applying this warrant police officers must be accompanied by an ASW and a doctor. Duration of this order is 72 hours.

Section 136 – police power to remove patients to a place of safety

This authorises the police to remove a person who appears to be suffering from mental disorder in a public place to a place of safety which is usually the A&E department of a hospital or a police station. The purpose of this is to enable further assessment by a doctor and an ASW and for any necessary arrangements for care and treatment to be made. Police officers should remain at the place of safety if required. Duration of this order is 72 hours.

Treatment orders

Section 3 – admission for treatment

The grounds for this longer-term order are that the patient is suffering from a specified mental disorder, which in practice means mental illness, severe mental impairment, mental impairment or psychopathic disorder. This should be of a nature or degree that makes it necessary to admit the person to hospital. A further stipulation is that such treatment is necessary for the health *or* safety of the patient *or* protection of others. Furthermore, in the case of a psychopathic disorder or mental impairment such treatment is likely to alleviate or prevent a deterioration in the patient's condition.

Duration of this order is 6 months in the first instance, renewable for a further 6 months and then annually subsequently. It requires authorisation by two doctors, one Section 12 approved. Application is by an ASW or nearest relative. The patient has a right of appeal to the MHRT in each period of detention. Discharge from this section can be by the RMO, nearest relative, hospital manager or the MHRT.

Section 7 – reception into guardianship

The purpose of this section is to place a patient who is at least 16 years old under the supervision of a guardian (usually the local social services authority or a named individual). The grounds for this may be as follows:

- The person is suffering from a mental disorder.
- It is necessary for the welfare of the patient or for protection of other persons.

Medical recommendation by two doctors, one approved, is required. Application is by an ASW or nearest relative. Duration of this order is 6 months, renewable for a further 6 months, then annually thereafter. The RMO, responsible social services authority or nearest relative have the power to discharge the person, who may appeal to the MHRT within the first 6 months, within the next 6 months and annually thereafter.

Guardianship powers

A guardianship application confers upon the authority or person named as a guardian the following powers:

- Power to require the patient to reside at a place specified
- Power to require the patient to attend at places, and times so specified, for the purpose of medical treatment, occupation, education or training
- Power to require access to the patient to be given, at any place where the patient is residing, to any registered medical practitioner, an ASW or other person so specified

Amy is a 25-year-old with a well documented diagnosis of schizophrenia and mild learning disability. Her full scale IQ was assessed to be 64. She lived with her parents and was dependent on them for appropriate supervision. She had poor community living skills and had limited literacy and numeric skills. She was vulnerable to exploitation without the support of her parents. Amy was admitted to hospital voluntarily when her mental health deteriorated. Although she came into hospital willingly, it quickly became apparent that she did not want to stay in hospital. On one occasion she absconded from the ward and was found by the police on a nearby motorway bridge. Amy was thus detained under Section 5/2 initially as she was already an in-patient. This was subsequently converted to Section 3 as she had a clear-cut diagnosis of schizophrenia in addition to her learning disability. Thus the category under which she was detained was 'mental illness', that is, schizophrenia. She needed treatment in hospital rather than further assessment followed by treatment. Thus Section 3 was considered to be more appropriate than Section 2. Whilst in hospital she appealed against her section and the MHRT consisting of a judge, a psychiatrist and a lay member upheld the section. For the tribunal Amy was supported by her own solicitor. Her parents also attended the tribunal and were supportive of Amy continuing to stay in hospital for further treatment. Amy was actively suicidal at the time making repeated self-harm attempts, for example trying to strangle herself with her tights. She thus spent a period of time in the psychiatric intensive care unit. After a stay of one year her condition finally stabilised with a change of medication. She has remained well after discharge and is fully complying with her care plan.

Admission and transfer of patients who have committed criminal offences

The Mental Health Act gives courts the power to:

- Remand an accused person to hospital for medical reports (Section 35)
- Remand an accused person to hospital for treatment (except murder cases) (Section 36)

- Make an interim hospital order on a convicted person for the purposes of assessing his or her suitability for a hospital order (Section 38)

Section 37 – hospital order
This is imposed by a court on a convicted offender who can be admitted to hospital for treatment under conditions similar to the civil provisions of Section 3. The duration is for 6 months, and again two medical recommendations are required, one from a Section 12 approved doctor. The crown court may in some cases make an additional order under *Section 41 – restriction order*, which restricts the person's discharge from hospital. Such an order can be for a specified period or without limit of time and is used with dangerous patients who have committed serious offences such as murder or arson or serious sexual offences.

Section 47 – transfer to hospital from prison
This authorises the Home Secretary to transfer a prisoner serving a sentence to a local NHS hospital or a special hospital. This can be with or without special restriction on discharge (Section 49), similar to Section 41 discussed above.

Medical treatments and second opinions

Section 58 – consent or second opinion
Under the Mental Health Act certain specified treatments require either the person to give consent or in the absence of this a second opinion from a second opinion approved doctor (SOAD). This rule applies to electroconvulsive therapy and continuation of medication after 3 months when a person is detained under Section 3.

Section 57 – consent and second opinion
For psychosurgery, which involves surgery affecting brain tissue and hormonal implants to reduce sex drive, both the patient's informed consent and a second opinion are required. Without this the treatment cannot go ahead.

Section 62 – urgent treatment
Such treatment that is immediately necessary to save life *or* prevent serious deterioration *or* is immediately necessary to alleviate serious suffering *or* represents the minimum interference to prevent violence or being a danger to self or others is allowed under common law. However, such treatment should not be hazardous or have any unfavourable, irreversible, physical or psychological consequences, for instance long-acting depot medication.

Role of the approved social worker (ASW)

Approved social workers are appointed by local social services for the purposes of discharging the functions conferred on them under the Mental Health Act. They:

- Interview the person
- Contact any relevant relatives/friends
- Ascertain whether there is a psychiatric history
- Consider any possible treatment alternatives to admission to hospital
- Make arrangements for compulsory admission to hospital
- Make any other necessary arrangements

Aftercare under supervision (supervised discharge)

Aftercare under supervision was introduced in April 1996 by the Mental Health (Patients in the Community) Act 1995. It is also referred to as *supervised discharge*.

This provision is designed to ensure that adequate aftercare is provided for patients who have been detained for treatment under Section 3 and who require suitable aftercare for their mental disorder in order to prevent a substantial risk of serious harm to self or others or of serious exploitation.

Patients must have a named community RMO who is the doctor in charge of their community treatment and a named CPA care coordinator. This order does not allow compulsory treatment in the community but allows a named professional to bring the patient to a hospital outpatient clinic for further assessment by a doctor. The provisions are similar to a guardianship order, but the health trust takes a lead in its administration.

Forensic aspects and risk

There has been a steady decline since the 1990s in the use of the Mental Health Act 1983 criminal provisions for offenders with learning disabilities. A minority of offenders with mild learning disability may be sent to prison due to lack of alternative provision. The prevalence of offending behaviour in those with learning disability is difficult to ascertain especially in those with mild learning disability, many of whom may not be in contact with any statutory service. Discrepancies in the definition of learning disability in research studies add to this uncertainty. Some of those with learning disability are vulnerable and easily led and more likely to get caught, thus coming into contact with the law (Lund 1990). Others are repeated offenders who take frequent impulsive risks. Prevalence of offending in the learning disabled population is low (around 1%) but the group with borderline learning disability is over represented in offender populations. Significant learning disability was identified in 2.3% of men sentenced and 6% of women (Gunn et al. 1991; Maden 1995). (For a full review of offending behaviour and learning disabilities see O'Brien 2002.)

West and Farrington's longitudinal prospective follow-up study of 411 working class boys born in 1953 found that those with convictions were more likely to have developmental difficulties, were poor academically at school, more hyperactive and impulsive at 10 years old and more likely to come from larger, poorer families where harsh, erratic discipline was used (Farrington 1985; Farrington and West 1993). Furthermore, chronic offenders could be predicted from a young age by behavioural problems, poverty, lower cognitive ability, a convicted parent and poor child-rearing methods (Farrington 1985).

Studies in hospital and court settings suggest an association between learning disability and sexual offences and arson. Possible reasons for association with sexual offences in those with borderline or mild learning disability could be lack of sexual knowledge, poor social skills, limited problem solving capacity, sex being thought of as a 'taboo' subject both by carers and those with the learning disability and in some cases inability to learn from past experiences or not knowing what is legally and morally right. Similar reasons apply to the association between arson and learning disabilities. The act of arson can also be the act of a powerless person resorting to extreme measures when their concerns are not heard or their needs not attended to. Lund (1990) found increased rates of violent crime and arson in his Danish study. People with severe learning disabilities who exhibit challenging behaviour in the form of severe physical aggression may not know that what they are is doing is illegal. Their intention may not be malicious although the result causes damage, distress or injury. Such acts usually do not lead to involvement of the police or the criminal justice system.

Mentally disordered offenders and court diversion schemes

There is an important provision of diversion from the criminal justice system of offenders who have learning disabilities or suffer from serious mental illnesses such as schizophrenia. People with learning disabilities are at an increased risk of wrongful conviction and false confessions (Gudjonsson 1992). The Reed report (Department of Health/Home Office 1994) recommends that 'court diversion and assessment schemes develop effective links with local learning disability teams and where possible team members contribute to schemes, possibly on a rota basis'.

The Police and Criminal Evidence Act 1984 (PACE)

When the police arrest a mentally disordered offender they are required to provide an 'appropriate adult' during the police interview. The appropriate adult has the important role of supporting the suspect with learning disability or mental illness and facilitating communication between the police, legal representatives and the suspect. The appropriate adult can be a relative or guardian but is most commonly a professional with training in this role and some knowledge of the suspect's disability.

The Criminal Procedure (Insanity) Act 1964 and Criminal Procedure (Insanity and Unfitness to Plead) Act 1991

The Criminal Procedure (Insanity) Act of 1964 allowed for the compulsory detention of those mentally disordered offenders who were unfit to plead at the time of their trial. In practice this led to unduly long periods of detention under secure conditions of offenders with learning disability without the benefit of a trial. Under the Act such persons could be detained in hospital until they regained fitness. This for some was an unattainable goal. The Act was revised and enacted in 1992, allowing for more flexibility when considering disposal options after finding someone to be unfit to plead. Thus a guardianship order, supervision and treatment order in the community and absolute discharge are other options available to the judge. For a person to be fit to plead he or she must demonstrate an understanding of court proceedings, that is, understand the nature of the charge and the difference between a plea of guilty and not guilty, be able to instruct a solicitor, challenge a juror and follow the evidence in court. Fitness to plead is assessed by two appropriately qualified doctors, one of whom should have special experience in the diagnosis and treatment of mental disorder. The evidence is presented to the court and the jury makes the final decision of whether a person is fit to stand trial.

Risk assessment

Assessing the risk a person poses to self or to others is a complex and difficult task. It is important to understand that there are no research instruments or scales that can predict with complete accuracy when a client will be dangerous to self or others. All professionals working within dual diagnosis services should have training in risk assessment and management. Risk assessment with an appropriate plan to manage and reduce the likelihood of the risk is an important part of the CPA. A multi-agency approach to risk assessment and management is recommended in clinical practice. However, the sad truth is that even with the best risk assessment practice, suicides and violent crimes will still occur. It is important that as professionals we use our knowledge to the best of our ability by carrying out a thorough assessment with a clearly formulated judgement of factors that may increase the risk, balanced by factors that are protective and reduce the likelihood of the risk occurring. Thus risk assessment is a dynamic process. Murphy et al. (2003) describe the development of a dynamic risk assessment and management system (DRAMS) to assess dynamic risk. They comment in their paper that there is considerable knowledge about static historical risk for future violent and sexual offending. This has resulted in a number of clinical tools for the assessment of risk in relation to violent and sexual offending, for example the Violence Risk Appraisal Guide (VRAG) (Quinsey et al. 1998) and the HCR-20 (Webster et al. 1997).

They divide risk factors into historical or actuarial risk factors and proximal or dynamic risk factors. The former will never change except perhaps to increase, while the latter vary constantly by the month, week or even the day. Hanson (2002) further divides dynamic factors into stable dynamic variables, which may be relatively unchanging although they may be amenable to treatment, for example poor anger control, and acute dynamic variables, which may change by the day or even by the hour, for example rages or level of provocation.

Effective Care Co-ordination policy (ECC)

The ECC policy guidelines provide a number of recommendations on risk assessment and management as follows (Department of Health 1999b):

- 'Risk assessment is an essential and on-going element of good mental health practice. Risk assessment is not, however, a simple mechanical process of completing a proforma. Risk assessment is an ongoing and essential part of the CPA process. All members of the team, when in contact with service users, have a responsibility to consider risk assessment and risk management as a vital part of their involvement, and to record those considerations.
- Risk cannot simply be considered an assessment of the danger an individual service user poses to themselves or others. Consideration also needs to be given to the user's social, family and welfare circumstances as well as the need for positive risk-taking. The outcome of such consideration will be one of the determinants of the level of multi-agency involvement.
- Risk assessment and risk management is at the heart of effective mental health practice and needs to be central to any training developed around the CPA. Staff must also consider the extent to which they might need support from colleagues, other services or agencies, especially when someone's circumstances or behaviour change unexpectedly.
- The *National Service Framework for Mental Health* (Department of Health 1999a) requires that care plans should specify the action to be taken in a crisis for all people on enhanced CPA. Crisis plans should set out the action to be taken based on previous experience if the user becomes very ill or his/her mental health is rapidly deteriorating.
- To reduce risk, the plan, as a minimum, should include the following information:
  — Who the user is most responsive to
  — How to contact that person
  — Previous strategies that have been successful in engaging the service user

This information must be stated clearly in a separate section of the care plan which should be easily accessible out of normal office hours.'

References

Department of Health (1999a) *A National Service Framework for Mental Health*. London: HMSO.

Department of Health (1999b) *Effective Care Co-ordination in Mental Health Services: Modernising the Care Programme Approach*. London: HMSO.

Department of Health (2001a) *Seeking Consent: Working with People with Learning Disabilities*. London: HMSO.

Department of Health (2001b) *Valuing People: A New Strategy for Learning Disability for the 21st Century*. London: The Stationery Office.

Department of Health (2002) *Keys to Partnership: Working Together to Make a Difference in People's Lives*. London: Department of Health.

Department of Health and Social Security (DHSS) (1971) *Better Services for the Mentally Handicapped*. Cmnd 4683. London: HMSO.

Department of Health and Welsh Office (1983) *Mental Health Act 1983 – Code of Practice*. London: HMSO.

Department of Health and Welsh Office (1999) *Code of Practice: Mental Health Act 1983*. Norwich: HMSO.

Department of Health/Home Office (1994) *Review of Health and Social Services for Mentally Disordered Offenders and Others Requiring Similar Services, Volume 7 – People with Learning Disabilities (Mental Handicap) or with Autism* (Chairman: Dr John Reed). London: HMSO.

Doll, E.A. (1965) *Vineland Social Maturity Scale*. Minnesota: American Guidance Service Incorporated.

Farrington, D.P. (1985) Predicting self-reported and official delinquency. In: D.P. Farrington and R. Tarling (Eds) *Prediction in Criminology*, pp. 150–173. Albany, New York: State University of New York Press.

Farrington, D.P. and West, D.J. (1993) Criminal, penal and life histories of chronic offenders: risk and protective factors and early identification. *Criminal Behaviour and Mental Health*, **3**, 92–523.

Fisher, T.W., Fowler, H. and Scarlet, J. (1978) *Normansfield Hospital: Report of a Committee of Inquiry* (Cmnd 7357). London: HMSO.

Fovargue, S. and Keywood, K. (2000) Participation in health care decision-making by adults with learning disabilities. *Mental Health Care*, **31** (10), 341–344.

Goffman, E. (1961) *Asylums – Essays on the Social Situation of Mental Patients and Other Inmates*. Garden City, New York: Doubleday.

Gudjonsson, G.H. (1992) *The Psychology of Interrogations, Confessions and Testimony*. Chichester: John Wiley.

Gunn, M. (1994) The meaning of capacity. *Medical Law Review*, **2**, 8–29.

Gunn, J., Maden, A. and Swinton, M. (1991) Treatment needs of prisoners with psychiatric disorders. *British Medical Journal*, **303**, 338–341.

Hanson, R.K. (2002) Introduction to the special section on dynamic risk assessment with sex offenders. *Sexual Abuse: A Journal of Research and Treatment*, **14**, 99–101.

Holland, A. (2003) Consent and decision making capacity. In: W. Fraser and M. Kerr (Eds) *Seminars in the Psychiatry of Learning Disability*, 2nd edition. London: The Royal College of Psychiatrists.

Howe Report (1969) *Report of the Committee of Enquiry into Allegations of Ill Treatment of Patients and Other Irregularities at the Ely Hospital, Cardiff*. Cmnd 3795. London: HMSO.

King's Fund Centre (1980) *An Ordinary Life*. London: King's Fund Centre.

Kramer, R. (2002) The Bournewood case. *Tizard Learning Disability Review*, **7**, 21–25.

Lund, J. (1990) Mentally disordered criminal offenders in Denmark. *British Journal of Psychology*, **156**, 726–731.

Maden, A. (1995) *Women, Prisons and Psychiatry*. London: Butterworth Heinemann.

Murphy, L., Smith, G., Murphy, D. et al. (2003) The development of a dynamic risk assessment and management system (DRAMS). Paper presented at The National Network for Learning Disability Nurses and The Foundation of Nursing Studies Conference, Manchester Metropolitan University, 14–15 July.

NHS Executive (1998) *Signposts to Success in Commissioning and Providing Health Services for People with Learning Disabilities*. London: The Stationery Office.

Nihira, K., Foster, R., Shellhaas, M. and Leland, H. (1974) *Adaptive Behaviour Scales*. Washington DC: American Association on Mental Retardation.

Nirje, B. (1969) The normalization principle and its human management implications. In: R.B. Kugel and W. Wolfensberger (Eds) *Changing Patterns in Residential Services for the Mentally Retarded*. Washington DC: President's Committee on Mental Retardation.

Nursing and Midwifery Council (1998a) *Guidelines for Records and Record Keeping*. London: NMC.

Nursing and Midwifery Council (1998b) *Guidelines for Mental Health and Learning Disability Nursing*. London: NMC.

Nursing and Midwifery Council (2001) *Position Statement on the Covert Administration of Medicines*. London: NMC.

Nursing and Midwifery Council (2002) *Code of Professional Conduct*. London: NMC.

O'Brien, G. (2002) Dual diagnosis in offenders with intellectual disability: setting research priorities: a review of research findings concerning psychiatric disorder (excluding personality disorder) among offenders with intellectual disability. *Journal of Intellectual Disability Research*, **46**, Suppl. 1, 21–30.

O'Brien, J. and Tyne, A. (1981) *Normalisation: A Foundation for Effective Services*. London: CMH.

Oswin, M. (1978) *Children in Long Stay Hospitals*. London: Spastics International Medical Publications.

Quinsey, V.L., Harris, J.T., Rice, M.E. and Cromier, C.A. (1998) *Violent Offenders: Appraising and Managing Risk*. Washington DC: American Psychological Association.

Ryan, J. and Thomas, F. (1995) *The Politics of Mental Handicap*. London: Free Association Books.

United Nations (1948) *Universal Declaration of Human Rights*. New York: United Nations.

United Nations (1971) *Declaration of the General and Specific Rights of the Mentally Retarded*. New York: United Nations.

Webster, C.D., Douglas, K.S., Eaves, D. and Hart, S.D. (1997) *HCR-20: Assessing Risk for Violence, Version 2*. Vancouver: Simon Fraser University Mental Health, Law and Policy Institute.

Wolfensberger, W. (1972) *The Principle of Normalisation in Human Services*. Toronto: National Institute on Mental Retardation.

Further reading

Ashman, L. and Duggan, L. (2004) Interventions for learning disabled sex offenders (Cochrane Review). In: *The Cochrane Library*, Issue 2. Chichester: John Wiley.

Department of Health (1999) *Effective Care Co-ordination in Mental Health Services –
Modernising the Care Programme Approach, a Policy Booklet*. London: Department of
Health.

Gelder, M., Gath, D. and Mayou, R. (1994) *Oxford Textbook of Psychiatry*. Oxford: Oxford
Medical Publications.

House of Commons Committee of Enquiry (1978) *Report of the Committee of Inquiry into
Normansfield Hospital*. London: HMSO.

Chapter 10

Service perspectives

Many people with dual diagnosis are often shifted between mental health and learning disability service structures in an effort to find appropriate services to meet their mental health needs. With this in view, this chapter will explore the service perspectives for people with dual diagnosis.

Key themes

- Care Programme Approach (CPA)
- Specialist versus mainstream mental health services
- Services for young people with learning disabilities
- Developing culturally sensitive services
- Developing partnership and collaboration

Introduction

The last two decades have seen a large reduction in the numbers of people with a learning disability living in hospital. Between 1980 and 1991 the numbers of hospital residents fell from 56 000 to 30 000, with a number of hospitals closing completely and approximately 70% of the remaining hospitals for people with learning disabilities scheduled for closure by the end of the millennium (Emerson and Hatton 1994). The policy guidelines stated in the White Paper *Valuing People* (Department of Health 2001) indicated the closure of all long-term hospitals for people with learning disabilities by the end of 2004, but the closure programme of the remaining hospitals is still continuing at the time of writing and is now scheduled to be completed by the end of 2006.

The shift in service provision from hospitals to the community has had a major impact on the range of services provided to this population. The development of community teams for people with learning disabilities (CTPLD) and multidisciplinary groupings of professional staff working at local level have contributed to the therapeutic services that are widely experienced by service users and their carers in the UK.

The National Health Service (NHS) and Community Care Act 1990 (Department of Health 1990) provided a strategic framework for the provision of all services in the community for people with a learning disability and their families. This Act united the principles through which care would be delivered between health and social services and encouraged statutory agencies to form partnerships with consumers, their representatives and with voluntary and independent sectors in order to provide a positive choice in the provision of services (Sines 1993). This gave birth to a new culture of locally based housing projects by a range of public, private and independent sectors. In addition to developments in residential provision, the Act also enabled people with a learning disability to directly access primary health care facilities.

The health needs of people with learning disabilities and the emphasis on primary care are gaining some attention. *The Health of the Nation* strategy for people with learning disabilities (Department of Health 1995) and the *Signposts for Success in Commissioning and Providing Health Services for People with Learning Disabilities* (NHS Executive 1998) stressed the requirement of generic and specialised services to meet the physical and mental health needs of these people. The White Paper *Valuing People* (Department of Health 2001) highlights the need to improve the health of people with learning disabilities through the introduction of health action plans and the appointment of health facilitators from each local CTPLD. In this context, learning disability nurses need to play a leading role in developing and shaping the nature of health care services for this population in partnership with primary care and mainstream health services.

Key issues in mental health services

In the UK, successive governments have inundated the field of mental health with policy initiatives. Indeed, social policy on mental health has been concerned more with mental illness, its management, amelioration and prevention than with mental health (Tudor 1996). The White Paper *Caring for People* (Department of Health 1989) identified four key principles of community care policy in its delivery of services:

(1) Flexibility and sensitivity
(2) Choice
(3) Minimum intervention
(4) Concentration on those with greatest need

The NHS and Community Care Act 1990 has had a major impact on mental health services in terms of the organisation and delivery of care. This legislation identified two key principles: identification of need and the provision of a package of care based on individual needs. The delivery of these individualised services fell on local authority, NHS mental health services and private and voluntary care providers. It is based on the notion that working within a mixed economy of care, care managers will be able to purchase the best available service based on the assessed needs of a person. This model based on free market economy failed to live up to its ideological expectations, due to the lack of a range of skilled service providers, lack of co-ordination between the agencies and lack of sufficient funding to meet individual needs.

The New Labour Government set out its vision of better mental health services in *Modernising Mental Health Services*, its new mental health strategy for England in December 1998 (Department of Health 1999c). This is placed in the context of wider NHS reforms and the strategy is based on providing a service 'in which patients and carers and the public are safe and where security and support is provided to all'. This resulted in the publication of a National Service Framework (NSF) for Mental Health in 1999 (Department of Health 1999a), which formed the agenda for modernising the mental health services in England. The NSF sets out 'seven standards' for mental health care – covering health promotion, primary care, access to services, acute and long-term community care in severe mental illness, services for carers and suicide prevention. These standards are as follows:

(1) Health and social services should promote mental health for all, working with individuals and communities, combating discrimination against people with mental health problems and promoting their social inclusion.
(2) Service users who contact their primary health care team with common mental health problems should have their mental health needs identified and assessed, and be offered effective treatments, including referral to specialist services for further assessment, treatment and care if they require it.
(3) Individuals with common mental health problems should be able to make contact around the clock with the local social services necessary to meet their needs and receive adequate care, and be able to use NHS Direct for first-level advice and referral on to specialist helplines or to local services.
(4) All mental health service users on the Care Programme Approach (CPA) should receive care that optimises engagement, prevents or anticipates crises and reduces risk. They should also have a copy of the written care plan which includes the action to be taken in a crisis by service users, their carers and their care co-ordinators, advises GPs how to respond if the service user needs additional help, and is reviewed regularly by the care co-ordinator; users should be able to access services 24 hours a day, 365 days a year.
(5) All service users who are assessed as requiring a period of care away from home should have timely access to an appropriate hospital bed, or an alternative bed or place, which is in the least restrictive environment consistent with the need to protect them and the public, and as close to home as possible. They should also have a copy of a written aftercare plan agreed on discharge, which sets out the care and rehabilitation to be

provided, identifies the care co-ordinator and specifies the action to be taken in crisis.

(6)   All individuals who provide regular and substantial care for a person on the CPA should have an assessment of their own caring, physical and mental health needs, repeated at least annually, and have their own written care plan, which is given to them and implemented in discussion with them.

(7)   Local health and social care communities should prevent suicide by:
— Promoting mental health for all, working with individuals and communities.
— Delivering high quality primary mental health care.
— Ensuring that everyone with a mental health problem can contact their local care services via the primary care team, a helpline and/or an A&E department.
— Ensuring that individuals with severe and enduring mental illness have a care plan that meets their specific needs, including access to services round the clock.
— Providing safe hospital accommodation for individuals who need it.
— Enabling individuals caring for someone with severe mental illness to receive the support that they need to continue to care.
— Supporting local prison staff in preventing suicides among prisoners.
— Ensuring that staff are competent to assess the risk of suicide among individuals at greatest risk.
— Developing local systems for suicide audit to learn lessons and take any necessary action.

For people with learning disabilities, the White Paper *Valuing People* states that most psychiatric disorders are common in people with learning disabilities and that the NSF for Mental Health, which applies to all adults of working age, is applicable to people with learning disabilities. In line with the seven standards identified in this NSF, the *Valuing People* document sets out the following seven areas for attention regarding people with learning disabilities in order to meet their mental health needs:

(1)   Mental health promotion materials and information about services should be provided in an accessible format for people with learning disabilities, including those from minority ethnic communities.

(2)   Strategies for improving access to education, housing and employment, which enhance and promote mental well-being, need to include people with learning disabilities and mental health problems.

(3)   Clear local protocols should be in place for collaboration between specialist learning disability services and specialist mental health problems.

(4)   For people with learning disabilities and mental health problems the health action plan should equate with the care plan. Care co-ordinators should have expertise in both mental health and learning disabilities. There should be close collaboration between psychiatrists in the relevant specialities.

(5) Specialist staff from learning disability services should if necessary provide support to crisis resolution/home treatment services or other alternatives to in-patient admission whenever possible.
(6) Each local service should have access to an acute assessment and treatment
resource for the small number of individuals with significant learning
disabilities and mental health problems who cannot appropriately be
admitted to general psychiatric services, even with specialist support.
(7) If admission to an assessment and treatment resource is unavoidable,
specialist staff should help patients understand and encourage them to
co-operate with treatment.

The NHS and Community Care Act 1990 introduced the process of care planning and care management in identifying individual needs and targeting the
services to meet these needs. The *Valuing People* document stresses the integration of the CPA and the care management process.

The Care Programme Approach (CPA)

The CPA was introduced in 1991 to provide a framework for effective mental
health care. The four key components of the CPA are:

(1) Systematic assessments of the health and social care needs of people
accepted into specialist mental health services
(2) The formulation of a care plan which identifies the health and social care
required from a variety of providers
(3) The appointment of a key worker or care co-ordinator to keep in close
touch with the service user and to monitor and co-ordinate care
(4) Regular reviews and where necessary agreed changes to the care plan

The CPA is a process with identifiable steps to plan and co-ordinate care for
people with mental illness. In the care of people with learning disabilities, the
care management principles and procedures based on the assessment of needs
and the development of a needs-led service have been in practice since 1993.
Hence it is essential that the CPA process should complement the existing care
management procedures and person-centred planning processes. For CPA to
be effective, professionals working in community teams, hospital based teams
and other settings must be in broad agreement with the criteria for eligibility
for the CPA (Roy 2000). The co-ordinator's knowledge and skills will undoubtedly influence the CPA process for a person with learning disability and
mental illness and hence it is essential that the co-ordinator has a sound
understanding of the mental health needs of people with learning disabilities,
awareness of needs assessment processes, knowledge of local services and
agencies and the ability to work in partnership with the individual, his/her
family and a range of service providers.

The Department of Health policy guidance on effective care co-ordination (ECC) in mental health services (Department of Health 1999b) aims to modernise the CPA further. It confirms the 'Government's commitment to the CPA as the framework for care co-ordination and resource allocation in mental health care'. ECC's primary stated aims are as follows:

- Integration of the CPA and care management
- Consistency in implementation of the CPA nationally
- To achieve a more streamlined process in order to reduce the burden of bureaucracy
- Proper focus on the needs of service users

ECC is particularly important for individuals whose care needs are complex, requiring the support of a number of agencies and services, and those who have so-called dual diagnosis, that is, a mental health problem associated with learning disability or a drug or alcohol problem. Individuals with mental health problems need support to access the full range of community supports required to promote their recovery and integration. Thus they may require assistance with housing, further education and appropriate leisure opportunities employment support and retraining and advice on disability benefits. People with learning disabilities *without* additional mental health needs may also require such supports to lead valued lifestyles. Thus when they suffer from additional mental disorders their needs become particularly complex, requiring collaboration between skilled multiprofessional teams from both learning disability and specialist mental illness services. The ECC policy introduced two levels of the CPA – standard and enhanced – throughout the country. The key worker is called the care co-ordinator. The key principles of CPA apply to both levels (standard and enhanced), that is, the right to a thorough assessment of the person's needs, the development of a care plan and regular review of that care by the professionals involved. For those individuals where there is only one professional providing ongoing help, this person is called the care co-ordinator. In addition the service users should be given the opportunity to sign the agreed care plan whenever possible and receive a copy of the plan.

The review of the care plan is seen as an ongoing process and at each review the date of the next review should be set and recorded. Furthermore, risk assessment and management is seen as an integral part of the ongoing CPA process. Care plans for the hospitalised severely mentally ill (for example those with schizophrenia and learning disabilities) should include urgent follow-up within one week of hospital discharge. Care plans for all those requiring enhanced CPA should include information on 'what to do in a crisis' and a contingency plan. Diverse needs related to gender, culture, ethnicity and sexuality must also be catered for. The needs of carers and children of parents with mental illness should also be actively assessed with plans to meet their needs.

The ECC policy identifies the following features of a truly integrated system of the CPA and care management:

- A single operational policy
- Joint training for health and social care staff
- One lead officer for care co-ordination across health and social care
- Common and agreed risk assessment and risk management processes
- A shared information system across health and social care
- A single complaints procedure
- Agreement on the allocation of resources and, where possible, devolved budgets
- A joint serious incident process
- One point of access for health and social care assessments and co-ordinated health and social care

The characteristics of people on standard CPA include those who:

- Require support or intervention of one agency or discipline or only low-key support from more than one agency or discipline
- Are able to self-manage their mental health problems
- Have an active informal support network
- Pose little danger to themselves or others
- Are likely to maintain appropriate contact with services

The characteristics of people on enhanced CPA include those who:

- Have multiple care needs, including those of housing, employment, etc., requiring inter-agency co-ordination
- Co-operate poorly with care agencies despite having multiple care needs
- Have contact with a number of agencies (including the criminal justice system)
- Require more frequent and intensive interventions, perhaps with medication management
- Have mental health problems co-existing with other problems such as substance misuse, learning disability or personality disorder
- Are at risk of harming themselves or others
- Are likely to disengage with services

It is important for practitioners and carers to understand that the CPA is a process of addressing the needs of a person with mental illness. The following case of Helen is an example of the CPA working well for a person.

Helen is a 23-year-old with chronic schizophrenia, mild learning disability, autistic disorder and a genetic diagnosis of 22q11 deletion syndrome (velo-cardio facial syndrome). She has had recurrent admissions to hospital which are usually precipitated by poor compliance with medication and the high degree of stress experienced by her mother, as the sole care provider, as a result of Helen's severe illness and behaviour problems. In view of her complex needs she is on enhanced CPA. Her care co-ordinator is a community psychiatric nurse from the specialist mental health service who works in close collaboration with the clinical psychologist from the community learning disability team. A social worker from the learning disability team has been involved in further planning of Helen's longer-term independent living needs. As part of this process the needs of her mother as the sole carer have also been assessed. Helen has been enabled to have regular respite at a local social services mental illness recovery facility. A team of support workers supervised by the care co-ordinator and the clinical psychologist have been commissioned to provide appropriate day care and support for further educational opportunities at a local college.

As with all other processes in care co-ordination, the CPA relies on the commitment of psychiatrics, nurses and other professionals and service providers. The CPA is applicable to a person with learning disabilities and mental illness accessing mainstream mental health services or a specialist learning disability service.

Mainstream vs specialist services

The White Paper *Valuing People* stresses the importance of people with learning disabilities using mainstream mental health and other services for meeting their mental health care needs. The policy directives aim at building inclusive services for people with learning disabilities and their carers. However, the experiences of many people with learning disabilities and their carers who have accessed mainstream mental health services are far from satisfactory. Hence, it is valid to ask the key question 'Is it an unrealistic expectation that the mainstream mental health services will be able to meet the mental health needs of people with learning disabilities?'.

One of most common uses of mainstream services by people with learning disabilities is the admission to general adult wards in mainstream mental health services. Many people with learning disabilities may find the general psychiatric wards too busy, chaotic and threatening, having come from quieter protected environments such as the family home or residential care. Nurses and other professionals on such wards do not usually have the training or skills to meet the needs related to the person's learning disability. They would expect each patient on the ward to quickly learn appropriate routines, for example meal times, times for medication rounds, days of ward rounds, days when occupational therapy activities are available and so on. A person with learning disability may have poor literacy skills and time sense, and thus be unable to read or tell the time.

The staff on the wards may be too busy with unpredictable acute emergencies to have the time to help the person with learning disability adjust to being on the ward. As a result people with learning disabilities may feel more confused due to the lack of individualised care and attention. They may feel more vulnerable in the general adult ward setting and be prone to abuse and exploitation. Admission of people with learning disabilities to mainstream mental health services may therefore take different routes (Chaplin and Flynn 2000), as follows:

- Admission to specified beds in general psychiatric wards with specially trained staff and cover by a learning disability consultant
- Admission to general psychiatric wards without specially trained staff but with consultant responsibility of a general psychiatrist in liaison with the community learning disability team
- Admission to a general psychiatric ward by default in the absence of any specialist service, where the general psychiatric team assumes all responsibility for care of the person whilst in hospital

The first model is a preferred option as there are specially trained staff who have sufficient understanding of the nature and manifestation of mental illness in people with learning disabilities. It is suggested that the use of this type of service in the mainstream sector can help to develop local expertise in mainstream services and reduce stigma (Chaplin and Flynn 2000).

Thiru (1994) provides an example of an integrated community service for people with learning disabilities in Lewisham, London. The community specialist psychiatric service (CSPS) for people with learning disabilities consists of a multidisciplinary team, which includes nurses with learning disability and mental health qualifications. Thiru explains the role of the community psychiatric nurse (CPN) for learning disabilities attached to this team and the effectiveness of that role in monitoring medication, setting up therapeutic interventions and management of care.

First and foremost in developing inclusive mental health services for people with learning disabilities, mainstream mental health services need the vision and commitment to make this a reality. Some of the reasons put forward for mental health services not being able to meet the needs of people with learning disabilities include:

- Lack of awareness and expertise of the nature and manifestation and the treatment modalities that can be applied to this population
- Poor knowledge and skills in detection and diagnosis of mental illness in people with learning disabilities
- Inadequate training for psychiatrists and also for nurses working in the mainstream mental health services
- Inadequate facilities (mainly beds) for accommodating people with learning disabilities
- Lack of a local strategy to foster partnership and joint working with learning disability and mental health services

The inability of the generic mental health services to adequately meet the mental health needs of people with learning disabilities has resulted in a number of private agencies capturing this market provision (Moss et al. 2000). These mainly consist of long-term residential provisions for people who may require medium secure services and ordinary residential services with additional staffing. After the closures of long-stay institutions, many NHS Trusts have also developed specialist assessment and treatment services and medium secure services to accommodate the needs of people with severe challenging behaviour and/or mental health disorders.

A rationale for specialised or a specialist mental health service for people with learning disabilities as part of the NHS has been put forward by Day (1993). In this paper he argues the need for specialist services because of (1) the requirement for specialist training and expertise to detect and diagnose mental illness in people with learning disabilities due to the atypical presentation and communication difficulties; (2) the unique nature of the highly specialised treatment techniques and the facilities required for the management of challenging behaviours; (3) the need for the modification of therapeutic interventions such as cognitive therapy, counselling and psychotherapy and subsequent evaluations with individuals or small groups; (4) the need for special regimes and careful monitoring of drug treatment in people with learning disabilities due to the high frequency of the side effects of medication and unusual responses in some people; (5) the need for special consideration due to the co-existence of physical disabilities and epilepsy which may complicate treatment and rehabilitation processes; and (6) offenders with learning disability being different from mentally disordered offenders, both in the nature and origins of their offending behaviour and their treatment needs. Day argues that specialised services increase staff competencies and skills, bringing the benefits of cumulative experience, which will ensure commitment to and ownership of assessment and treatment processes.

The two main models of specialist services for people with learning disabilities and mental health disorders consist of:

- Residential services, which may consist of in-patient and outpatient services and in some cases long-term residential provision for people with enduring mental health needs
- Services that are linked to the community teams for people with learning disabilities or community mental health teams

The Reed report (Department of Health 1994) on the review of services for mentally disordered offenders recommended the following:

- Services should emphasise prevention in order to reduce the impact of the offending behaviour on the individuals concerned, their carers and on society.

- Community services need to liaise with the police, courts, prisons, probation, mental illness and forensic psychiatry services, local authorities and other relevant organisations involved with offenders.
- Service provision should include differing levels of security, less than that provided by special hospitals, and thus reduce inappropriate admissions to special hospitals.
- Ready access should be available to special in-patient regional units for evaluation and treatment, both in the short term and in the long term.
- Specially skilled staff who are well trained and well supported are required.
- Such work is stressful so there should be effective managerial and professional support to staff and staffing levels may need to be augmented at times of crises.

There is a growing evidence base for specialist services for people with learning disability and mental illness. Kwok (2001) describes the development of a specialised in-hospital psychiatric unit that was designed to provide mental health care for people with learning disabilities. A hospital-based system with multidisciplinary input and strong community linkage was adopted and funded almost entirely by redistributing existing resources. Since the service came into operation, the responses received from patients, carers and other service providers in the community have been highly favourable. The author claims the project is important because it signifies a major step forward in diversifying the health care of people with learning disabilities.

Minnen et al. (1997) investigated the effectiveness of hospital and outreach treatment of patients with learning disability and psychiatric disorders. A total of 50 patients were randomly assigned to either the hospital treatment or the outreach treatment group. The outcome measures included psychiatric symptoms, family burden costs and hospital admissions. At all endpoints the two groups were equivalent with regard to psychiatric symptoms, and the burden on carers did not increase significantly during the outreach treatment. It is concluded that outreach treatment represents an effective and efficient alternative to hospitalisation for patients with mental retardation and psychiatric disorders. The evaluation of an in-patient treatment service in Leicester (Trower et al. 1998) over a 2 year period suggested that the specialist in-patient unit was able to meet the needs of adults with learning disability and psychiatric problems through short-term in-patient assessment and treatment.

Holden and Neff (2000) studied the impact of intensive versus outpatient mental health interventions in a dual diagnosis clinic on the hospitalisation rate and length of stay of 28 adults with learning disabilities and severe psychiatric disorder selected on the basis of frequent use of mental medical and social services. Charts were reviewed for the 12 month period before and after referral to the programme in order to compare service utilisation. A single pre-test and post-test design with no control group was employed. Correlated tests comparing the pre- and post-test programme number of hospitalisations indicated significant decreases in hospitalisations and lengths of stay after programme entry, which may result in significant reductions in hospital costs.

Young people with learning disabilities

Young people with learning disabilities and mental health problems in the UK fall between a number of health care providers, including child and adolescent mental health services, specialist learning disability services, primary care and childrens' services. A description of the full range of services for such young people is not available in the literature. McCarthy and Boyd (2002) studied the extent of use of specialist health services during adolescence by a group of young people with learning disabilities and mental health problems over a period of time. They studied 80 young people with learning disabilities, who were examined in childhood and adolescence for psychiatric and behaviour disorder. These individuals were interviewed again in early adult life for the presence of psychiatric and behaviour disorders. A key finding of this study is that the majority of young people with persistent challenging behaviour from adolescence or childhood psychiatric disorder received no specialist mental health professional input during the transition period into adult services.

The report of the Royal College of Psychiatrists (1998) into the psychiatric services for children and adolescents with learning disabilities suggests the need for a range of therapies (diagnosis, adjustment counselling, family work, specialised individual therapies including medication) to be carried out in conventional outpatient facilities. The report also suggests the need for a residential or in-patient setting either for crisis management, through assessment and effective treatment, or where the person cannot be contained within his or her home or by the family.

The report of the enquiry into the mental health needs of young people with learning disabilities (Foundation for People with Learning Disabilities 2002) recommends that mainstream mental health services should develop the resources and expertise to respond to young people in providing inclusive services. The report highlights the need for retaining specialist services and their valuable support to mainstream services for young people with most complex needs. The report stresses the key areas of service development for young people with learning disabilities and mental illness, which should include the following:

- *Clear pathways into services*: families are often unclear about the range of services available for children and young people with learning disabilities and ways of accessing these services. There is a need for transparency and clarity in the referral mechanisms to paediatricians, the child and adolescent mental health services (CAMHS) and services within the learning disability sector.

- *Transition into adult services*: young people with learning disabilities face serious gaps in services at the point of transition from school or college to adult services. There should be an agreed protocol for effective services between learning disability and mental health services for young people at the point of transition.
- *More resources*: this is crucial in providing effective mental health services. The lack of adequate financial and human resources to meet the mental health needs of young people results in creating more crisis interventions that are not person or family friendly and also results in the young person being admitted to specialist provisions far away from the family. There is an urgent need for knowledgeable and skilled professionals and support staff to care for young people with learning disabilities and mental illness.
- *A multidisciplinary approach*: the need for multidisciplinary working is stressed, but its visibility in practice is lacking. Professionals and agencies need to work together with families to recognise the needs of young people and to identify and implement helping models and practices. There is a need to come up with imaginative models of help services that may not fit the traditional therapeutic service structures.

The need for better services for children and young people is echoed in a report to the Department of Health in 2000 by the Young Minds organisation (www.youngminds.org.uk) on child and adolescent mental health services (Tunnard 2000). This report identifies the need for mental health support in schools, for children and young people in care, multiprofessional core teams, help for frontline staff, better access to specialist services and for strategic planning and better links between child and adult services. The essence of support for the mental health of young people with or without learning disabilities can be summed up in a simple quote from this report:

'Children and young people need to be cared for by adults who look after their emotional needs as well as their physical and intellectual needs: children and young people need to learn how to make friends and have good relationships with people around them; they need resilience to cope with difficulties and disappointment; and they need a belief of their own self-worth and that of others.' (Tunnard 2000)

Mental health promotion for young people with learning disabilities should be seen as a collaborative venture between the family, primary care services, child and adolescent mental health services, schools and other organisations such as the Connexions service. Connexions is the Government's support service for young people aged 13 to 19. The service provides advice, support and access to personal development opportunities to aid the transition to adulthood and working life.

Types of services

The structure of services for people with learning disabilities and mental illness may take different forms. A full description of all the possible service structures is not possible here, but some of the most common forms followed by many of the services in the UK are explored.

Assertive outreach teams (AOTs)

Assertive outreach teams is the term given to the deployment of a multi-disciplinary team to provide outreach assessment and interventions for people living in the community. The aim is to assess, treat and maintain people in their own homes. The AOT will be involved in intense case management and is intended to work with those individuals who are found to be difficult to manage by other services. AOTs can help people with learning disability and mental illness by providing help and support in their own living environment. For example, Thiru (2002) describes the working of an AOT in Hackney, London, and Porter and Sangha (2002) provide a detailed account of the working of an AOT in Oxfordshire.

Mental health specialists attached to community teams

This may take the form of learning disability nurses or other professionals who are specifically employed within community teams for people with learning disabilities (CTLD) to work with individuals suspected or diagnosed as having mental illness and their families and carers. One example is a model implemented in Oxfordshire by the Learning Disability NHS Trust in 1996 where learning disability nurses were attached to community teams. These specialist nurses or other professionals will be part of the community team and hence should be able to accept referrals directly from the team. They should carry a small caseload (not more than 10 people at a time) so that they are able to work with individuals, their families or carers over a longer time. They will conduct initial assessments (such as screening for mental illness) and report to the CTLD for further assessment and intervention procedures that may need to be implemented. They may be able to prevent crisis developing for the individual or the family through their initial assessment and care planning. Moreover, the assessments may help in highlighting the level of stress of the family or carers and its potential to develop into a crisis in the future. This will help the team to identify and implement clear action plans through these specialist nurses and professionals and evaluate the impact of their roles on a case-by-case basis.

Liaison workers

Services are also introducing liaison workers, who liaise with learning disability, primary care and mainstream mental health services. The key aim here is to help a person with learning disability and mental health problems to use the mainstream services as far as possible by offering specialist input into the mainstream mental health service.

In-patient assessment and treatment services

A specialist in-patient unit to assess and treat people with learning disabilities who experience mental illness is an essential part of any service structure for people with learning disabilities. This facility will be able to provide assessment and treatment that may not be possible in the person's own living environment, that is, the person's family home or residential home. Moreover, people who need to be sectioned under the Mental Health Act for assessment and/or for treatment will require safe settings with well-trained and confident multi-disciplinary staff. This service should provide a therapeutic environment for those requiring intense assessment and treatment for a relatively short period of time.

Developing culturally sensitive services

All service providers should view developing inclusive services for people with learning disabilities from different cultural backgrounds as a priority. The White Paper *Valuing People* shows that the needs of people from black and minority ethnic communities are often overlooked (Department of Health 2001). People with learning disabilities and their families in general face barriers in accessing ordinary services and marginalisation in society; people with learning disabilities from black and minority ethnic communities often face double discrimination due to their disability and their cultural or religious background; and needless to say, these people face triple discrimination if they also experience additional mental health problems. Research in relation to services for minority ethnic communities has highlighted a number of problems relating to access to such support. A key factor here is knowledge and awareness of existing services. In a study of young people with learning disabilities and mental health needs from a South Asian community in Bradford (Raghavan et al. 2005), carers were eloquent in stating their case of the lack of awareness of services for their son or daughter:

> 'People don't know about them (services), where to go, where not to go and how to get help.'
>   'I don't know . . . we don't know how to get help and I have been here for 26 years.'
>   'No one has ever told me about the different types of help I could get . . . so don't know what's out there.'

Statements like these from family carers highlight the lack of awareness of existing services and how to access these services. The lack of staff who could speak the same language as the carer, the cultural inappropriateness of existing services in terms of activities, staff provision and diet, and racial discrimination within services have all contributed to low take-up and poor service development (Baxter 1998; Hatton et al. 1998, 2000).

Mir et al. (2001) argue that attempts to provide culturally sensitive services do not always address individuals' needs, however, and may simply group people together because they are from the same ethnic group (or sometimes based on colour) without due regard to different needs relating to age, nature of disability or diverse interests. People in such groups may feel uncomfortable if they do not have much in common with other group members. The range of activities that some specialist support groups offer can be limited and if there is no progression to other provision this can lead to underachievement.

The Race Relations (Amendment) Act 2000 states that services should end discrimination and promote equality and it suggests that all organisations should have a race equality scheme setting out their plan to address cultural diversity and equality within services. The strategy document *Inside Outside: Improving Mental Health Services for Black and Minority Ethnic Communities in England* (Department of Health 2003) highlights the inequalities of mental health care for black and minority ethnic groups. It is suggested that these inequalities should be tackled by focusing on the cultural capability of the organisation or improving the capacity of the organisation in providing high quality service, irrespective of the ethnic or cultural background of the people using the service.

Malek (2004) argues that delivering culturally sensitive services requires recognition of cultural beliefs and practices at both practical and therapeutic levels. In providing culturally sensitive services, Malek highlights a broad range of activities such as:

- A policy framework that supports a culturally sensitive response at all levels.
- Data collection on minority ethnic communities generally and the number of people from minority ethnic groups attending each service.
- Research into theory and practice issues necessary to deliver culturally sensitive practice.
- Collaboration with ethnic and other agencies to ensure that the needs of specific ethnic groups are understood and addressed.
- Education for staff and the wider community, which tailors explanations for mental health and ill-health so as to reduce the fear and stigma associated with mental illness in minority ethnic groups.
- Administrative structures that support the delivery of culturally sensitive practice.
- Training of clinical and administrative staff to respond sensitively when dealing with people from a range of cultures.
- Assessment and intervention procedures that take into account the culturally defined needs of the person, his or her family and the community.

A key component of a culturally sensitive service is its visibility to the local ethnic community. Language is a key factor in encouraging access to services by people from minority ethnic communities and hence information about the available services should be provided in all the languages spoken in the community. It is essential to realise that offering culturally sensitive services is not just the collection of data on ethnicity (which is a tick box exercise), but having a broader understanding of the diverse cultures in the community, their cultural and religious needs and learning about appropriate ways of responding to these needs.

Partnership and collaboration

People with dual diagnosis present unique challenges to health professionals, in terms of both diagnosis and the provision of appropriate therapeutic services. Considering the nature of dual diagnosis, people with learning disability and mental health disorder will require specialised services (Day 1993). The Mansell report (Department of Health 1993) suggests that service planning and delivery for people with learning disability and mental health disorder should be highly individualised to meet the widely differing needs of these people. However, in reality, people with dual diagnosis are often shuffled between mental health and learning disability service sectors, with neither of them taking full responsibility for appropriate therapeutic services (Naylor and Clifton 1993; Turnbull 1996). The continued argument over who owns the case has on many occasions led to loose arrangements in planning and delivery of therapeutic services for this population (Turnbull 1996).

People with dual diagnosis constantly face barriers and stigma in accessing and use of mainstream mental health services, which is working against the principles of promoting inclusive services in our society. People with dual diagnosis are often 'made to do' by slotting them into existing service structures. As we have seen in this book, people with learning disabilities and mental health disorders have complex needs which require individually negotiated and arranged opportunities and solutions. This calls for collaborative working within and across agencies planning and commissioning therapeutic services.

The White Paper *Valuing People* (Department of Health 2001) emphasises the need for people and organisations to work in partnership to achieve the aim of inclusive services for people with learning disabilities. Anchoring on inclusion, rights and choices for people with learning disabilities, the *Keys to Partnership* document (Department of Health 2002) states that:

'the main reason for people to work together is to make sure that people with learning disabilities can have socially inclusive lives. We should work on this with a person centred approach. This means that we should really be listening and learning about what people with learning disabilities and their families want and need. It means that people who use services and their families are at the centre of any decisions that are made about their lives and about the help that they need to live the way they want to.' (p. 3)

There needs to be a constructive dialogue between professionals, commissioners and service-providing agencies in meeting the individual needs of people with dual diagnosis living in a range of service sectors through active partnership and collaboration. Cole (2002) highlights the plight of people with dual diagnosis in obtaining the appropriate services that they require and identifies 12 key factors in developing effective service structures for this population. These consist of:

(1)   Person-centred planning approaches
(2)   Individualised purchasing
(3)   Targeted skilled community support
(4)   Links with primary care
(5)   Flexible funds for flexible support
(6)   Positive leadership
(7)   Partnership developments across services and specialisms
(8)   Specific support for 'vulnerable adults'
(9)   A local place for people to stay, with intensive support, in a crisis
(10) Working with and developing existing providers
(11) Evidence to support developments
(12) Fostering mutual support to reduce isolation and build strength

In general, service structures for people with learning disabilities are diverse consisting a of a number of providers in the health and social service partnership, voluntary and private sectors. The challenge for services is to provide the right kind of help at the right time for people with dual diagnosis in the context of multi-agency service provision. People with dual diagnosis require flexible and person-centred care necessitating working across agencies in the spirit of developing and sustaining innovative service models that are inclusive and sensitive to these people's cultures and beliefs. This is a challenge for commissioners and service providers, requiring them to work together with mutual respect and shared vision to create better services for people with learning disabilities and mental health disorders.

Conclusion

People with dual diagnosis receive a bad deal from mainstream mental health services. Services for people with learning disabilities and mental health disorders need to take account of their individual needs in the commissioning process. The health and social policy governing the care of people with mental health problems and people with learning disabilities advocates partnership and collaborative working with all service providers and commissioners. The challenge is for nurses and other professionals in the learning disability and mental health sectors to develop the willingness to work together in reducing the health inequalities experienced by people with dual diagnosis.

References

Baxter, C. (1998) Learning difficulties. In: S. Rawaf and V. Bahl (Eds) *Assessing Health Needs of People from Minority Ethnic Groups.* London: Royal College of Physicians/ Faculty of Public Health Medicine.

Chaplin, R. and Flynn, A. (2000) Adults with learning disability admitted to psychiatric wards. *Advances in Psychiatric Treatment*, **6**, 128–134.

Cole, A. (2002) *Include Us Too: Developing and Improving Services to Meet the Mental Health Needs of People with Learning Disabilities.* London: IAHSP, Kings College.

Day, K. (1993) Mental health services for people with mental retardation: a framework for the future. *Journal of Intellectual Disability Research*, **37**, 7–15.

Department of Health (1989) *Caring for People: Community Care in the Next Decade and Beyond.* Cmnd 849. London: HMSO.

Department of Health (1990) *The National Health Service and Community Care Act.* London: HMSO.

Department of Health (1993) *Services for people with Learning Disabilities and Challenging Behaviour or Mental Health Needs* (Chairman: Professor J. Mansell). London: HMSO.

Department of Health (1994) *Review of Health and Social Services for Mentally Disordered Offenders and Others Requiring Similar Services: People with Learning Disabilities (Mental Handicap) or with Autism* (Chairman: Dr John Reed), Vol. 7. London: HMSO.

Department of Health (1995) *The Health of the Nation: A Strategy for People with Learning Disabilities.* London: HMSO.

Department of Health (1999a) *National Service Framework for Mental Health. Modern Standards and Service Models.* London: Department of Health.

Department of Health (1999b) *Effective Care Coordination in Mental Health Services: Modernising the Care Programme Approach.* London: Department of Health.

Department of Health (1999c) *Modernising Mental Health Services: Safe, Sound and Supportive.* London: Department of Health.

Department of Health (2001) *Valuing People: A Strategy for Learning Disability for the 21st Century.* London: The Stationery Office.

Department of Health (2002) *Keys to Partnership: Working Together to Make a Difference in People's Lives.* London: Department of Health.

Department of Health (2003) *Inside Outside: Improving Mental Health Services for Black and Minority Ethnic Communities in England.* London: National Institute for Mental Health in England.

Emerson, E. and Hatton, C. (1994) *Moving Out: Relocation from Hospital to Community.* London: HMSO.

Foundation for People with Learning Disabilities (2002) *Count Us In: The Report of the Committee of Enquiry into Meeting the Mental Health Needs of Young People with Learning Disabilities.* London: Foundation for People with Learning Disabilities.

Hatton, C., Azmi, S., Caine, A. and Emerson, E. (1998) Informal carers of adolescents and adults with learning difficulties from South Asian communities: family circumstances, service support and carer stress. *British Journal of Social Work*, **28** (6), 821–837.

Hatton, C., Akram, Y., Shah, R., Robertson, J. and Emerson, E. (2000) *Supporting South Asian Parents of a Child with Severe Disabilities*. Lancaster: Institute of Health Research, Lancaster University.

Holden, P. and Neff, J. (2000) Intensive outpatient treatment of persons with mental retardation and psychiatric disorder: a preliminary study. *Mental Retardation*, **38**, 27–32.

Kwok, H.W.M. (2001) Development of a specialised psychiatric service for people with learning disabilities and mental health problems: report of a project from Kwai Chung Hospital, Hong Kong. *British Journal of Learning Disabilities*, **29**, 22–25.

Malek, M. (2004) Meeting the needs of minority ethnic groups in the UK. In: M. Malek and C. Joughin (Eds) *Mental Health Services for Minority Ethnic Children and Adolescents*. London: Jessica Kingsley.

McCarthy, J. and Boyd, J. (2002) Mental health services for young people with intellectual disability: is it time to do better? *Journal of Intellectual Disability Research*, **46**, 250–256.

Minnen, A. Hoogduin, C.A.L. and Broekman, T.G. (1997) Hospital versus home treatment for people with mental retardation and serious mental illness: a case controlled study. *Acta Psychiatrica Scandinavica*, **95**, 515–522.

Mir, G., Nocon, A. and Ahmad, W. with Jones, L. (2001) *Learning Difficulties and Ethnicity: Report to the Department of Health*. London: Department of Health.

Moss, S. Bouras, N. and Holt, G. (2000) Mental health services for people with intellectual disability: a conceptual framework. *Journal of Intellectual Disability Research*, **44**, 97–107.

Naylor, V. and Clifton, M. (1993) People with learning disabilities – meeting complex needs. *Health and Social Care in the Community*, **1**, 343–353.

NHS Executive (1998) *Signposts for Success in Commissioning and Providing Health Services for People with Learning Disabilities*. London: Department of Health.

Porter, I. and Sangha, J. (2002) Reaching out. *Learning Disability Practice*, **5**, 18–21.

Raghavan, R., Waseem, F., Small, N. and Newell, R. (2005) *Making Us Count: Identifying and Improving Mental Health Support for Young People with Learning Disabilities*. London: Foundation for People with Learning Disabilities.

Roy, A. (2000) The Care Programme Approach in learning disability psychiatry. *Advances in Psychiatric Treatment*, **6**, 380–387.

Royal College of Psychiatrists (1998) *Psychiatric Services for Children and Adolescents with a Learning Disability*. Council Report CR70. London: Royal College of Psychiatrists.

Sines, D. (1993) Nursing people with learning disabilities; new directions. *British Journal of Nursing*, **2**, 510–514.

Thiru, S. (1994) Focal point. *Nursing Times*, **90** (12), 62–64.

Thiru, S. (2002) Assertive outreach. *Learning Disability Practice*, **5**, 10–13.

Trower, T. Treadwell, L. and Bhaumik, S. (1998) Acute in-patient treatment for adults with learning disabilities and mental health problems in a specialised admission unit. *British Journal of Developmental Disabilities*, **44**, 20–29.

Tudor, K. (1996) *Mental Health Promotion: Paradigms and Practice*. London: Routledge.

Tunnard, J. (2000) *Report for the Department of Health on Child and Adolescent Mental Health Services*. www.youngminds.org.uk.

Turnbull, J. (1996) Your case or mine. *Nursing Times*, **92** (23), 62–63.

Further reading

Department of Health (1989) *Needs and Responses*. London: HMSO.

Department of Health (1991) *Assessment Systems and Community Care*. London: HMSO.

Department of Health (1991) *Care Management and Assessment: Practitioner's Guide*. London: HMSO.

Department of Health (1994) *Stephen Dorrell's MENCAP Speech/Statement on Services for People with Learning Disabilities*, 25 June. London: HMSO.

Department of Health and Social Security (1979) *Report of the Committee of Inquiry into Mental Handicap Nursing and Care* (Chair: Mrs P. Jay) Vols I and II, Cmnd 7468-I, 7468-II. London: HMSO.

Felce, D. (1996) Changing residential services: from institutions to ordinary living. In: P. Mittler and V. Sinason (Eds) *Changing Policy for People with Learning Disabilities*. London: Cassell.

King's Fund Centre (1980) *An Ordinary Life*. London: King's Fund Centre.

Rapley, M. and Ridgway, J. (1998) 'Quality of life' talk and the corporatisation of intellectual disability. *Disability and Society*, **13**, 451–471.

Welsh Office (1983) *The All-Wales Strategy for the Development of Services for Mentally Handicapped People*. Cardiff: Welsh Office.

Appendix 1

Assessment tools

Assessment is a key aspect of planning appropriate care for people with dual diagnosis. As the nature and manifestation of mental illness in people with learning disabilities is a complex process, the assessment process can be enhanced by the use of standardised measures. Some of the key assessment tools that are applicable to people with dual diagnosis are described below.

Screening tools

The Psychopathology Instrument for Mentally Retarded Adults (PIMRA)

The Psychopathology Instrument for Mentally Retarded Adults (PIMRA) developed by Matson (1988) is a rating scale that can be completed quickly by third-party informants and interviewers with psychiatric training and by self-report. This scale based on DSM-III classification has 56 items organised into eight separate scales allowing for assessment of the absence of psychopathology as well as seven specific disorders defined in accordance with DSM-III: schizophrenia, depression, somatoform disorders, psychosexual disorders, adjustment disorders, anxiety disorders and personality problems.

PIMRA is available in two different versions: a rating-by-other form, to be filled in by a person who has a good knowledge of the person with learning disability, and a self-report form, to be filled in by the person with learning disability him- or herself and to be used only with people with mild learning disability. It can be used either for an early screening of the person at risk or for the formulation of a diagnosis. Cut-off scores are available for diagnostic purposes and have been used in some prevalence studies (Iverson and Fox 1989). PIMRA has shown adequate to good reliability for items and scale totals and good internal consistency (Sturmey 1993).

- Iverson, J.C. and Fox, R.A. (1989) Prevalence of psychopathology among mentally retarded adults. *Research in Developmental Disabilities*, **10**, 77–83.
- Matson, J.L. (1988) *The PIMRA Manual*. Orland Park, Los Angeles: International Diagnostic Systems.

- Sturmey, P. (1993) The use of DSM and ICD diagnostic criteria in people with mental retardation: a review of empirical studies. *Journal of Nervous and Mental Disease*, **181**, 38–41.

The Reiss Screen for Maladaptive Behaviour

The Reiss Screen for Maladaptive Behaviour (Reiss 1988) is a 38 item psychometric instrument designed for use in screening large populations in order to identify those persons who need further evaluation as to the presence of a psychiatric or behavioural disorder. It is a rating scale designed to be completed by carers, teachers or supervisors who know the clients well enough to make valid reports of their behaviour and mental state. It was developed in the USA and studies using this screening instrument are largely based on the US population of people with learning disabilities (Reiss 1990; Sturmey et al. 1995).

The Reiss Screen contains 38 statements, each signifying a problem in the lives of people with learning disability. Each item refers to a psychiatric symptom or behavioural category, rather than to a specific observable behaviour. A multiple-criteria rating system is used to reflect the multiple dimensions along which psychopathology is judged. The behaviours are considered to be psychopathological based on their frequency of occurrence, the circumstances under which they occur, the suffering they cause for the subject and society, and the intensity of the behaviour.

The Reiss Screen requires raters to use all these criteria in judging whether a psychiatric symptom is currently 'no problem', 'a problem' or 'a major problem' in the life of the person being evaluated. The *Reiss Screen Manual* suggests that teachers, caretakers and work supervisors who know the person well enough to report the behaviour accurately could make the ratings. The Reiss Screen recommends the use of two or more raters for each participant. The purpose of obtaining two ratings rather than one is to assess sample behaviour from a broad range of circumstances in order to have test scores that express the opinions of two people rather than the opinion of a single person (Reiss 1988).

Reiss (1997) suggests that each item on the Reiss Screen is presented in three parts: the name of the symptom (for example hallucinations); a non-technical definition (for example experiencing things that are not there); and common behavioural examples (hearing voices, hearing sounds, having visions or strange bodily sensations, etc.). According to Reiss, the purpose of the definitions and common behavioural examples is to improve understanding of the items on the part of the raters, who in the majority of cases are not mental health professionals, but unqualified carers.

The Reiss Screen provides three screening methods to be used in combination (Reiss 1997). According to Reiss the purpose of using three methods is to minimise the number of false negatives by providing three ways in which a person could be referred for professional evaluation.

Scoring of the Reiss Screen

The scoring system of the Reiss Screen consists of: (1) seven scale scores, (2) six special maladaptive behaviour item scores, and (3) the 26 item total score. (For screening purposes a total score is computed with 26 items from the test, which is known as the 26 item total score.)

The seven scale scores are based on the results of a factor analysis of a national sample of 305 people. Each scale has five items, with some items counting on more than one scale. The seven scales are: aggressive disorder, psychosis, depression (behavioural signs), depression (physical signs), avoidant disorder, dependent personality disorder and paranoia. Reiss added autism as another scale after factor analysis. He suggests that the item content of the autism scale should be based primarily on the diagnostic signs of autism.

In addition to the seven scale scores, six special maladaptive behaviours are scored. The six maladaptive behaviour items include drug abuse, overactivity, self-injury, sexual behaviour, suicidal tendencies and stealing. According to Reiss (1997), a person rated by the carer as suicidal should be referred for psychiatric or psychological evaluation regardless of any other information, including total score and diagnostic status.

A 26 item total score is computed to identify whether a person has tested positive or negative for mental health disorder using the cut-off score. Reiss recommends this as people with severe disorders show symptoms character-istic of a variety of disorders. For example, people with severe psychosis tend to show some symptoms of anxiety disorder, and people with severe panic attacks tend to show some symptoms of psychosis. Reiss suggests that the 26 item total score may be viewed as a measure of the severity of the psychopa-thology. The more severe the case of psychopathology, the greater the number of symptoms present and the higher the Reiss Screen total score. The total score is the sum of the scores for the 26 items used in calculating the seven scale scores. Each of the scoring criteria (seven scale scores, six special items and the total score) has a cut-off point. According to the *Reiss Screen Manual*, a person with learning disability is said to test 'positive' for dual diagnosis if any of the three categories (seven scale scores, six special maladaptive item score and the 26 item total score) is at or above the cut-off points.

- In the 26 item total score, a person is said to test positive for dual diagnosis if he or she scores 9 or above in this category.
- In the seven scale scores, a person is said to test positive for these items if he or she scores 4.5 or above in each of the categories.
- In the special maladaptive behaviour item scores, a person is said to test positive for these items if he or she scores 1.5 or above on each of the items.

In order to screen a person with learning disability for mental health disorder, the 26 item total score is used as the overall score.

Interpretation of test results

A positive test result means that the subject is likely to need a mental health service (Reiss 1988) and should be referred to mental health professionals in order to determine the validity of test results and for further investigation of his or her mental state.

- Reiss, S. (1988) *The Reiss Screen for Maladaptive Behaviour*. Ohio: IDS Publishing Corporation.
- Reiss, S. (1990) Assessment of a man with a dual diagnosis. *Mental Retardation*, **30**, 1–6.
- Reiss, S. (1997) Comments on the Reiss Screen for Maladaptive Behaviour and its factor structure. *Journal of Intellectual Disability Research*, **41**, 346–354.
- Sturmey, P., Burcham, K.J. and Perkins, T.S. (1995) The Reiss Screen for Maladaptive Behaviour: its reliability and internal consistencies. *Journal of Intellectual Disability Research*, **39**, 191–195.

The PAS-ADD checklist

Moss et al. (1998) developed the PAS-ADD checklist (Psychiatric Assessment Schedule for Adults with a Developmental Disability) as a screening tool from the PAS-ADD interview schedule (Moss et al. 1993). The aim of the checklist is to screen people with learning disabilities who experience mental illness. Hence, the central purpose of the checklist is to discriminate as sensitively and accurately as possible between those who have significant mental health problems and those who do not (Moss et al. 1998).

The checklist consists of a life-events checklist and 29 symptom items scored on a four-point scale. Moss et al. (1998) suggest that the items are worded in everyday language, making the checklist suitable for use by individuals who do not have a background in the assessment of psychopathology.

The broad areas of the checklist encompass:

- Appetite and sleep
- Tension and worry
- Phobias and panics
- Depression and hypomania
- Obsessions and compulsions
- Psychoses
- Autism

Scoring of the PAS-ADD checklist

The scoring of the checklist is simple and self-explanatory:

(1) Total score I: affective or neurotic disorder (maximum possible score = 28; threshold = 6)

(2) Total score II: possible organic condition (maximum possible score = 8; threshold = 5)

(3) Total score III: psychotic disorder (maximum possible score = 6; threshold = 2)

Any person scoring 1 or more above the three thresholds is identified as having a potential psychiatric disorder, which should be further investigated. For anyone scoring near to the threshold, but not exceeding it, the recommendation is that he or she should be monitored regularly and completely.

- Moss, S., Patel, P., Goldberg, D., Simpson, N. and Lucchino, R. (1993) Psychiatric morbidity in older people with moderate and severe learning disability. 1. Development and reliability of the patient interview (PAS-ADD). *British Journal of Psychiatry*, **163**, 471–480.
- Moss, S., Prosser, H., Costelleo, H., et al. (1998) Reliability and validity of the PAS-ADD checklist for detecting disorders in adults with intellectual disability. *Journal of Intellectual Disability Research*, **42** (2), 173–183.

Assessment of Dual Diagnosis (ADD)

The Assessment of Dual Diagnosis (ADD) constructed by Matson and Bamburg (1998) provides information on diagnoses, developing treatment plans and evaluating treatment outcomes. The ADD administration manual suggests that it was developed as a measure to screen for symptoms typically reported in research and clinical practice as problematic for individuals with mild or moderate mental retardation. Matson and Bamburg claim that the items for the ADD derived from DSM-IV (American Psychiatric Association 1994) and from previously published studies with this population (Enfield and Tonge 1995). The dimensions of the scale are rated in terms of specific frequency, duration and severity levels rather than simply endorsing the presence or absence of behaviours or subjective estimates of symptom severity.

The ADD is a 79 item psychopathology instrument representing 13 diagnostic categories. They include: (1) mania, (2) depression, (3) anxiety, (4) post-traumatic stress disorder, (5) substance abuse, (6) somatoform disorders, (7) dementia, (8) conduct disorder, (9) pervasive developmental disorder, (10) schizophrenia, (11) personality disorders, (12) eating disorders and (13) sexual disorders. Ratings are on a scale of 0 to 2 for each dimension. By acquiring ratings across each of these domains, the ADD depicts the extent to which a particular behaviour or symptom is problematic.

- American Psychiatric Association (1994) *Diagnostic and Statistical Manual of Mental Disorders (DSM-IV)*. Washington DC: APA.
- Enfield, S.L. and Tonge, B.J. (1995) The developmental behaviour checklist: the development and validation of an instrument for the assessment of behavioural and emotional disturbance in children and adolescents with

mental retardation. *Journal of Autism and Developmental Disorders*, **25**, 81–104.

- Matson, J.L. and Bamburg, J. (1998) Reliability of the Assessment of Dual Diagnosis (ADD). *Research in Developmental Disabilities*, **20**, 89–95.

Psychiatric interview schedules

Psychiatric Assessment Schedule for Adults with a Developmental Disability (PAS-ADD)

PAS-ADD is a semistructured psychiatric interview standardised for people with learning disabilities. This interview schedule is based on Present State Examination (PSE) (Wing et al. 1974) and the Schedules of Clinical Assessment in Neuropsychiatry (SCAN) (WHO 1992). The PAS-ADD produces research diagnosis and involves present-state interviewing of the patient, followed by a similar interview with a key informant. This interview schedule can be applied to detect symptoms and to produce a diagnosis. The authors of PAS-ADD claim that this schedule can be used for the psychiatric assessment of individuals whose linguistic ability does not permit a clinical interview.

- Wing, J.K., Cooper, J.E. and Sartorius, N. (1974) *Measurement and Classification of Psychiatric Symptoms: An Instruction Manual for the PSE and CATEGO Program.* Cambridge: Cambridge University Press.
- World Health Organization (1992) *Schedules of Clinical Assessment in Neuropsychiatry.* Geneva: WHO.

The Mini PAS-ADD

The Mini PAS-ADD is derived from the full PAS-ADD interview schedule. The Mini PAS-ADD is not an interview schedule. It provides a framework for an individual or a team of individuals to collect together relevant information on psychiatric symptomatology, which is available without the need for interviewing. The Mini PAS-ADD is aimed at case identification, rather than full ICD-10 diagnostic evaluation (Prosser et al. 1998).

This instrument comprises a list of 86 psychiatric symptoms and generates a series of sub-scores on: depression, anxiety and phobias, mania, obsessive–compulsive disorder, psychosis, unspecified disorder (including dementia) and pervasive developmental disorder (autism). All items are rated on a four-point scale of severity.

- Prosser, H., Moss, S., Costello, H., Simpson, N., Patel, P. and Rowe, S. (1998) Reliability and validity of the Mini PAS-ADD for assessing psychiatric disorders in adults with intellectual disability. *Journal of Intellectual Disability Research*, **42** (4), 264–272.

Practice Guidelines for the Assessment and Diagnosis of Mental Health Problems in Adults with Intellectual Disability

This is not an assessment tool, but provides comprehensive guidelines for the assessment of mental illness in people with learning disabilities. It lists the assessment tools available for people with learning disabilities (Deb et al. 2001).

- Deb, S., Mathews, T., Holt, G. and Bouras, N. (2001) *Practice Guidelines for the Assessment and Diagnosis of Mental Health Problems in Adults with Intellectual Disability*. Brighton: Pavilion.

Needs assessment

The Learning Disability version of the Cardinal Needs Schedule (LDCNS)

The LDCNS provides a systematic process of needs assessment covering 23 areas of functioning using a battery of standardised instruments (see Chapter 5 and Raghavan et al. 2004).

- Raghavan, R., Marshall, M., Lockwood, L. and Duggan, L. (2004) Assessing the needs of people with learning disabilities and mental illness: development of the Learning Disability version of the Cardinal Needs Schedule. *Journal of Intellectual Disability Research*, **48**, 25–37.

The Camberwell Assessment of Needs for adults with Developmental and Intellectual Disability (CANDID)

CANDID provides the systematic assessment of needs covering 22 areas of functioning (see Chapter 5 and Xenitidis et al. 2000).

- Xenitidis, K., Thornicroft, G., Leese, M., et al. (2000) Reliability and validity of the CANDID – a needs assessment instrument for adults with learning disabilities and mental health problems. *British Journal of Psychiatry*, **176**, 473–478.

Appendix 2
Genetic syndromes related to mental health

Prader–Willi syndrome

In 1956 Prader, Labhart and Willi discovered a rare genetic disorder affecting 1 in 15 000.

Clinical features: Neonatal hypotonia and poor feeding, hypogonadism, small stature, small hands and feet. Typical dysmorphic facial appearance with a small bifrontal diameter, a triangular mouth and almond-shaped eyes. Strabismus and scoliosis also reported. Cognitive impairment usual. Gross hyperphagia leading to obesity from early childhood (Beadsmore et al. 1998).

Genetic information: Deletion on the long arm of chromosome 15 of paternal origin, may be caused by a paternal gene mutation (Deb 1997).

Behavioural phenotype: Maladaptive behaviours include temper tantrums, self-injury, impulsiveness, lability of mood, inactivity, repetitive speech, impulsive talk, stubbornness and physical aggression directed at others and property. Various types of sleep disturbance have been reported (Deb 1997). Reports of skin picking resulting in infection (Clarke et al. 1996) and non-food obsessions and compulsions (Dykens et al. 1996).

Reported associations with mental disorders: Mainly case reports. Clarke et al. (1998) reported six cases with psychotic symptoms. Beardsmore et al. (1998) reported 25 cases of affective psychosis. Verhoeven et al. (1998) reported six cases of cycloid psychosis.

Williams syndrome

This occurs in 1 in 55 000 live births.

Clinical features: Distinct facial appearance, early feeding difficulties, failure to thrive, growth retardation, joint laxity, hyperacusis, renal and cardiovascular abnormalities. Majority suffer moderate to severe learning disability.

Genetic information: Microdeletion at the site of the elastin gene on chromosome 7 (Ewart et al. 1993).

Behavioural phenotytpe: Deficits in visuo-spatial abilities and gross and fine motor skills. Language abilities better, with superficially fluent social language and precocious vocabulary, but with poor turn taking and topic maintenance skills and limited comprehension (Udwin et al. 1998). Behaviour problems include overactivity, restlessness, irritability, preoccupations and obsessions, poor social relationships with peers and overfriendliness.

Reported associations with mental disorders: Reported high levels of anxiety and fearfulness. Infants show abnormal attachment behaviour with indiscriminate affection and anxiety. Further research is required for links to mental disorders.

Fragile X syndrome

This is a familial X-linked disorder first reported by Martin and Bell (1943). It is the most common inherited cause of learning disability, affecting 1 in 1200 males and 1 in 2000 to 2500 females.

Clinical features: Characteristic facial appearance including a large forehead, long nose, prominent chin and large ears. There may be eye abnormalities and genital anomalies. Other features include hyperextensible joints, flat feet, inguinal and hiatus hernia, enlarged aortic root and mitral valve prolapse.

Genetic information: Area of constriction near the end of the long arm of the X chromosome. Gene recently discovered (FMR1).

Behavioural phenotype: Hyperarousal, restlessness, poor concentration, aggression, ritualistic behaviour and other autistic features, stereotyped behaviour and mannerisms, unacceptable eccentric habits and antisocial behaviour reported. Deficits in social interaction, non-verbal communication, social withdrawal, delayed echolalia, repetitive speech and hand flapping.

Reported associations with mental disorders: Case reports suggest a high prevalence of anxiety disorders (Bregman et al. 1988) and social anxiety (Hagerman and Sobesky 1989). Psychotic problems, shyness, anxiety, schizotypal features and intermittent depressive disorder said to be significantly higher in female carriers (Freund et al. 1992).

Rett syndrome

Rett (1966, cited in Lindberg 1991) described 22 cases of a syndrome affecting girls exclusively because it is fatal for male fetuses (Deb 1997). Prevalence 1 in 10 000 to 15 000. Learning disability usually severe to profound.

Clinical features: Babies develop normally up to 18 months to 2 years. Then stereotyped motor movements develop involving hands and fingers, in the form of hand flapping and wringing movements. There is a slowing of development. Some features resemble autism and hence there is a chance of misdiagnosis. Epilepsy develops by the age of 4 or 5, and spasticity of limbs also develops at this time.

Genetic information: No gene discovered although some suspect a dominant gene on the X chromosome.

Behavioural phenotype: Self-injurious behaviour, sleep problems, hyperventilation, mood changes and anxiety reported. Sudden noises, some types of music, strange people or places, or excessive activity in the proximity of the child seem to precipitate episodes of anxiety (Deb 1997).

Reported associations with mental disorders: No specific associations reported. Anxiety and mood changes have been reported, but further research is needed to explore links with mental health disorders.

Down's syndrome

This is the most common cause of learning disability, affecting 1 in 1000 live births. Greater risk with advancing maternal age at conception.

Clinical features: Short stature with round skull. Eye signs include typical 'mongoloid slope' of the palpebral fissures. Prone to develop cataracts prematurely. Some congenital abnormalities of the internal organs, for example atrial or ventricular septal defects, oesophageal atresia, congenital dilatation of the colon, umbilical and inguinal hernia. People with Down's syndrome develop hypothyroidism, repeated chest infections and sleep apnoea.

Genetic information: 95% of cases due to trisomy 21, 4% translocation and 1% mosaicism (Deb 1997).

Behavioural phenotype: Cheerful, affectionate, humorous, amiable, music loving and good at mimicry, but also stubborness.

Reported associations with mental disorders: Studies show nearly 45% of adults with Down's syndrome over the age of 45 develop dementia (Zigman et al. 1995).

References

Beadsmore, K., Dormamn, T., Cooper, S.-A. and Webb, T. (1998) Affective psychosis and Prader–Willi syndrome. *Journal of Intellectual Disability Research*, **42** (6), 463–471.

Bregman, J.D., Leckman, J.F. and Ort, S.I. (1988) Fragile X syndrome: genetic predisposition to psychopathology. *Journal of Autism and Developmental Disorders*, **18**, 343–354.

Clarke, D.J., Boer, H., Chung, M.C., Sturmey, P. and Webb, T. (1996) Maladaptive behaviour in Prader–Willi syndrome in adult life. *Journal of Intellectual Disability Research*, **40**, 159–165.

Clarke, D., Boer, H., Webb, T., et al. (1998) Prader–Willi syndrome and psychotic symptoms: 1. Case descriptions and genetic studies. *Journal of Intellectual Disability Research*, **42** (6), 440–450.

Deb, S. (1997) Behavioural phenotypes. In: S. Reed (Ed.) *Psychiatry in Learning Disabilities*. London: W.B. Saunders.

Dykens, E.M., Leckman, J.F. and Cassidy, S.B. (1996) Obsessions and compulsions in Prader–Willi syndrome. *Journal of Child Psychology and Psychiatry*, **37**, 995–1002.

Ewart, A.K., Morris, C.A., Atkinson, D., et al. (1993) Hemizygosity at the elastin locus in a developmental disorder, Williams syndrome. *Nature Genetics*, **5**, 11–16.

Freund, L.S., Reiss, A.L. and Hagerman, R.J. (1992) Chromosome fragility and psychopathology in obligate female carriers of the fragile X chromosome. *Archives of General Psychiatry*, **49**, 54–60.

Hagerman, R.J. and Sobesky, W.E. (1989) Psychopathology in fragile X syndrome. *American Journal of Orthopsychiatry*, **59**, 142–152.

Lindberg, B. (1991) *Understanding Rett Syndrome*. Toronto: Hogrefe and Huber.

Martin, J.P. and Bell, J. (1943) A pedigree of mental defect showing sex linkage. *Journal of Neurology and Psychiatry*, **6**, 154–157.

Udwin, O., Howlin, P., Davies, M. and Mannion, E. (1998) Community care for adults with Williams syndrome: how families cope and the availability of support networks. *Journal of Intellectual Disability Research*, **42**, 238–245.

Verhoeven, W.M.A., Curfs, L.M.G. and Tuinier, S. (1998) Prader–Willi syndrome and cycloid psychoses. *Journal of Intellectual Disability Research*, **42** (6), 455–462.

Zigman, W., Schupf, N., Haveman, M. and Silverman, W. (1995) *Epidemiology of Alzheimer's Disease in Mental Retardation: Results and Recommendations from an International Conference*. Washington DC: American Association on Mental Retardation.

Index